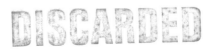

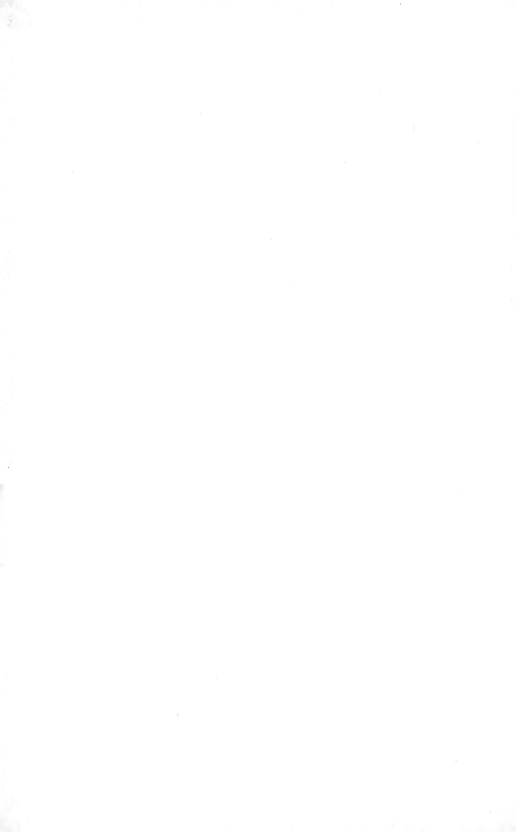

DRUG EDUCATION LIBRARY

CAFFEINE

by Hal Marcovitz

LUCENT BOOKS

An imprint of Thomson Gale, a part of The Thomson Corporation

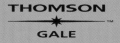

THOMSON
™
GALE

Detroit • New York • San Francisco • San Diego • New Haven, Conn.
Waterville, Maine • London • Munich

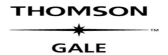

THOMSON

GALE

™

Produced by OTTN Publishing, Stockton, N.J.

© 2006 Thomson Gale, a part of The Thomson Corporation.

Thomson and Star Logo are trademarks and Gale and Lucent Books are registered trademarks used herein under license.

For more information, contact
Lucent Books
27500 Drake Rd.
Farmington Hills, MI 48331-3535
Or you can visit our Internet site at http://www.gale.com

LIBRARY OF CONGRESS CATALOGING-IN-PUBLICATION DATA

Marcovitz, Hal.
  Caffeine / by Hal Marcovitz.
    p. cm. — (Drug education library)
  Includes bibliographical references and index.
  ISBN 1-59018-863-2 (hard cover : alk. paper)
  1. Caffeine—Physiological effect—Juvenile literature. 2. Caffeine habit—Health aspects—Juvenile literature. I. Title. II. Series.
  RC567.5.M37 2006
  615'.785—dc22
                    2005036214

Printed in China

CONTENTS

Foreword

The development of drugs and drug use in America is a cultural paradox. On the one hand, strong, potentially dangerous drugs provide people with relief from numerous physical and psychological ailments. Sedatives like Valium counter the effects of anxiety; steroids treat severe burns, anemia, and some forms of cancer; morphine provides quick pain relief. On the other hand, many drugs (sedatives, steroids, and morphine among them) are consistently misused or abused. Millions of Americans struggle each year with drug addictions that overpower their ability to think and act rationally. Researchers often link drug abuse to criminal activity, traffic accidents, domestic violence, and suicide.

These harmful effects seem obvious today. Newspaper articles, medical papers, and scientific studies have highlighted the myriad problems drugs and drug use can cause. Yet, there was a time when many of the drugs now known to be harmful were actually believed to be beneficial. Cocaine, for example, was once hailed as a great cure, used to treat everything from nausea and weakness to colds and asthma. Developed in Europe during the 1880s, cocaine spread quickly to the United States where manufacturers made it the primary ingredient in such everyday substances as cough medicines, lozenges, and tonics. Likewise, heroin, an opium derivative, became a popular painkiller during the late nineteenth century. Doctors and patients flocked to American drugstores to buy heroin, described as the optimal cure for even the worst coughs and chest pains.

As more people began using these drugs, though, doctors, legislators, and the public at large began to realize that they were more damaging than beneficial. After years of using heroin as a painkiller, for example, patients began asking their doctors for larger and stronger doses. Cocaine users reported dangerous side effects, including hallucinations and wild mood shifts. As a result, the U.S. government initiated more stringent regulation of many powerful and addictive drugs, and in some cases outlawed them entirely.

A drug's legal status is not always indicative of how dangerous it is, however. Some drugs known to have harmful effects can be purchased legally in the United States and elsewhere. Nicotine, a key ingredient in cigarettes, is known to be highly addictive. In an effort to meet their bodies' demands for nicotine, smokers expose themselves to lung cancer, emphysema, and other life-threatening conditions. Despite these risks, nicotine is legal almost everywhere.

Other drugs that cannot be purchased or sold legally are the subject of much debate regarding their effects on physical and mental health. Marijuana, sometimes described as a gateway drug that leads users to other drugs, cannot legally be used, grown, or sold in this country. However, some research suggests that marijuana is neither addictive nor a gateway drug and that it might actually benefit cancer and AIDS patients by reducing pain and encouraging failing appetites. Despite these findings and occasional legislative attempts to change the drug's status, marijuana remains illegal.

The Drug Education Library examines the paradox of drugs and drug use in America by focusing on some of the most commonly used and abused drugs or categories of drugs available today. By discussing objectively the many types of drugs, their intended purposes, their effects (both planned and unplanned), and the controversies surrounding them, the books in this series provide readers with an understanding of the complex role drugs and drug use play in American society. Informative sidebars, annotated bibliographies, and organizations to contact lists highlight the text and provide young readers with many opportunities for further discussion and research.

THE WORLD'S MOST POPULAR DRUG

Each year, Americans consume approximately 2.4 billion gallons of tea, 6.3 billion gallons of coffee, 15.3 billion gallons of soft drinks, and 3.1 billion pounds of chocolate. These products share a common ingredient: caffeine, a stimulant that affects the brain and central nervous system.

Consumption of caffeine is far from an American phenomenon. In many countries, the use of coffee and tea is a part of the national culture. Caffeine-bearing crops like coffee or cacao beans, kola nuts, and tea leaves dominate the economies of numerous countries in South and Central America, Africa, and Asia. Although worldwide consumption figures are impossible to estimate, there is no doubt that caffeine is the most commonly used drug in the world.

The chemical structure of caffeine is $C_8H_{10}N_4O_2$, meaning it is composed of carbon, hydrogen, nitrogen, and oxygen atoms. Caffeine is a substance that occurs naturally in plants. Botanists believe it is a product of evolution; the substance is poisonous to certain insects, so it protects the plant from being damaged by bugs. There are about sixty plants that produce caffeine, most of which grow in tropical zones.

Caffeine is generally considered a beneficial drug because of its many positive attributes. Each morning millions of people rely on caffeine's stimulating effects by beginning their days with a cup of coffee or tea. Some writers, artists, and other creative people insist that caffeine helps clear their minds and enhance their powers of concentration. Similarly, some athletes have found that consuming caffeine shortly before workouts or competitions helps them perform better. Caffeine has also been found to help people lose weight, and may help prevent certain kind of cancers, as well as diabetes and other diseases.

Nevertheless, like other drugs, caffeine does have addictive qualities and can cause negative health effects when abused. Excess caffeine consumption can lead to sleeping problems,

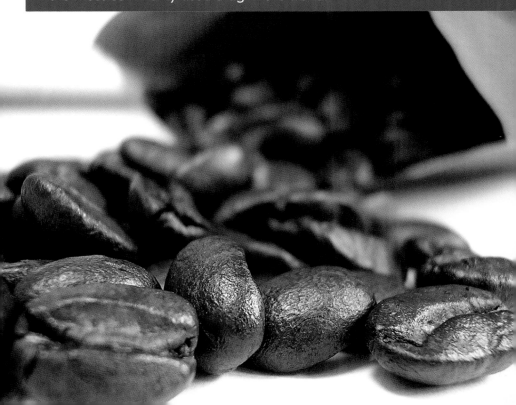

These coffee beans are among many plant beans or seeds that naturally contain caffeine. This mostly beneficial substance is the most commonly used drug in the world.

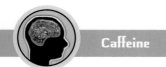
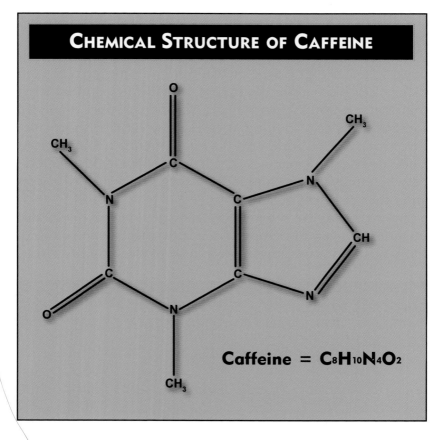

CHEMICAL STRUCTURE OF CAFFEINE

Caffeine = $C_8H_{10}N_4O_2$

feelings of anxiousness or jitteriness, muscle aches, and increased heartbeat, among other problems.

According to Bennett Alan Weinberg, co-author of the book *The World of Caffeine: The Science and Culture of the World's Most Popular Drug,*

> Caffeine is a drug in every sense of the word. You know, the word "drug" is used in different ways. It can be used to refer to something that affects your system physically. It can be something that affects your mind. It can be something that's addictive. Caffeine is a drug in all of these senses. It is an addictive, psychoactive substance that has profound effects on the mind and body.[1]

Caffeine Serving Sizes

The amount of caffeine that people ingest can vary greatly, depending on the caffeinated products they prefer. Coffee is generally considered to be the most heavily caffeinated beverage; the amount of caffeine in an eight-ounce cup generally varies from about 80 to 150 milligrams. (Some brands of coffee are significantly stronger than this average; for example, eight ounces of Starbucks coffee contains more than 240 milligrams of caffeine.) The caffeine level of the average instant coffee is slightly lower than that of regular coffee, generally ranging from about 65 to 125 milligrams.

An eight-ounce cup of tea contains about fifty milligrams of caffeine. However, the amount of caffeine can vary greatly, depending on the blend of tea leaves used. Some teas may have as much as one hundred milligrams of caffeine, while green tea contains less caffeine—about thirty milligrams per cup. (Herbal teas are naturally decaffeinated; the herbs used in these teas do not contain caffeine.)

Coca-Cola and Pepsi, two of the most popular soft drinks, contain thirty-four and thirty-seven milligrams of caffeine, respectively. The caffeination of these drinks occurs because their formula includes kola nuts, which naturally contain caffeine, for flavor. Many soft drinks not flavored with kola nuts, such as 7-Up, Sprite, and most ginger ales and root beers, contain no caffeine. There are other soft drinks that do not use kola nuts in their formulas but do contain caffeine. Some manufacturers add the drug to help with flavoring as well as to make the drinker feel more energetic. Mountain Dew, for example, is flavored with citrus rather than with kola nuts. Caffeine is added to the beverage during manufacturing because its bitter taste is believed to counteract the very sweet citrus, making the drink more palatable. A twelve-ounce serving of Mountain Dew contains about fifty-five milligrams of caffeine, making it one of the more heavily caffeinated soft drinks. Other artificially caffeinated soft drinks include Dr. Pepper, Mr. Pibb, Shasta, and Sunkist.

In recent years, so-called "energy drinks" have become popular in the United States and other countries. These drinks often have high caffeine levels, similar to that of a cup of coffee. An eight-ounce can of Red Bull, for example, contains about eighty milligrams of caffeine, while a twelve-ounce can of Jolt Cola contains about seventy-one milligrams of caffeine.

Chocolate and other cocoa products have a fraction of the caffeine found in coffee, tea, and soft drinks. A cup of hot cocoa, for example, contains just ten milligrams of caffeine, while an ordinary Hershey's chocolate bar contains twelve milligrams of caffeine. The small amounts of caffeine in chocolate exist because caffeine is part of the chemical makeup of the cacao bean, which is used in the manufacture of chocolate.

Caffeine also is available in tablet form in any pharmacy, supermarket, or health food store. It is sold as an "alertness aid" under such brand names as Vivarin and NoDoz. The caffeine these products contain is approximately the equivalent of two cups of average-strength coffee (about two hundred milligrams). Caffeine is also a common ingredient in some painkillers; Excedrin, for example, contains about sixty-five milligrams of caffeine per capsule.

Safe in Moderate Doses

Because caffeine can be found in so many products, Americans begin regularly consuming the drug at an early age. Most people begin drinking soft drinks, iced teas, hot cocoas, and other caffeinated beverages when they are young, then add coffee and tea when they reach high school or college. Fortunately, most physicians see no harm in caffeine as long as it is consumed in moderate doses. The amount of caffeine required for a fatal overdose is almost impossibly high.

Caffeine is not safe for everyone, however. For example, in recent years medical professionals have warned pregnant women to avoid caffeine because it can cause miscarriages.

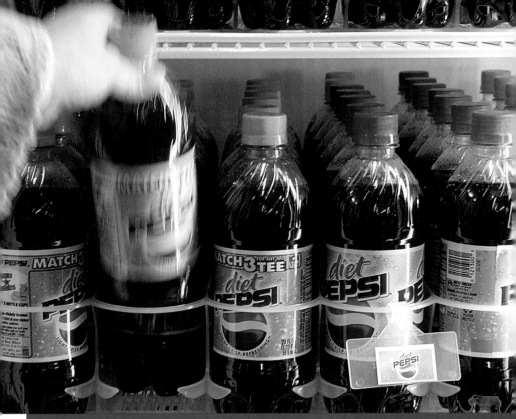

Caffeinated sodas are among the most popular drinks in the United States today, particularly among young people. The amount of caffeine varies depending on the brand of drink.

Doctors also believe certain dietary supplements, in which caffeine is combined with the herb ephedra, can cause dangerous or fatal effects. For a time, the U.S. Food and Drug Administration banned this combination.

After thousands of years of use, caffeine remains one of the least understood of all drugs. Scientific research continues to turn up new facts about caffeine. While some of the new discoveries are alarming, others indicate that caffeine is a beneficial drug that may have significant promise as a disease fighter.

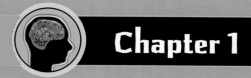

Chapter 1

CAFFEINE THROUGH THE AGES

According to legend, an Ethiopian goatherd named Kaldi discovered the energizing effects of coffee beans when the animals in his flock refused to sleep after eating the leaves and berries of a plant they found while foraging in the mountains. In fact, the next morning when Kaldi led the goats back to the grazing area, the animals immediately returned to the same plants. According to this tale, Kaldi found that when he ate the berries himself, he felt a rush of energy, and he soon told others about the miraculous plant.

Whether or not this story is true, some scientists believe Stone Age humans ate coffee berries and beans (which contain most of the plant's caffeine) for energy. And throughout history, humans have ingested many other plants that contain caffeine. The Chinese began using the leaves of the bush Camellia sinensis to brew tea before 600 B.C. At around the same time in central Mexico, the Mayans started using the beans of the cacao tree to make chocolate (although their version was very different from the chocolate eaten today.) Other caffeine-containing substances include kola nuts, which were commonly chewed by the indigenous peoples of

West Africa and Indonesia, and the guarana plant, which was believed by certain tribes in South America to have healing and strength-renewing properties.

The Spread and Influence of Tea

The first caffeinated beverage for which humans have written records is tea. In China, generally considered the birthplace of tea drinking, recorded consumption of the beverage dates back nearly 3,000 years. According to one Chinese legend, tea was developed by accident, when the ancient emperor

This rare color photograph from the early 20th century shows a Chinese man standing in front of tea bushes. The Chinese have brewed tea for thousands of years.

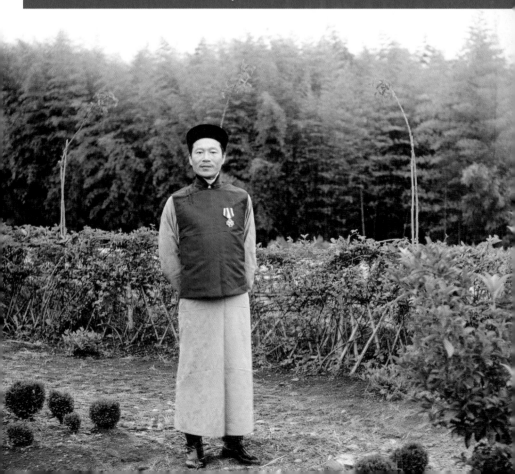

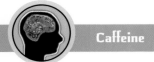
Shennong was preparing a cup of hot water to drink. Some leaves fell into the cup, changing the color of the water and giving off a pleasant smell. The curious emperor took a sip

England Discovers Tea

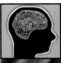
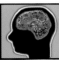

The English can thank Queen Catherine of Braganza for introducing tea to their empire. The Portuguese-born princess married King Charles II in 1662. Her large dowry included a chest of tea grown in India. Catherine served the tea at court, and drinking tea quickly became a popular custom.

In 1663, the English poet Edmund Waller wrote the verse "Of Tea Commended by Her Majesty," honoring Catherine for presenting the drink to her subjects. The poem mentions

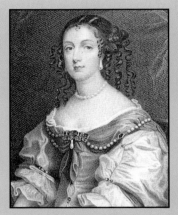

Catherine of Braganza (1638–1705) is credited with introducing tea to England.

the benefits of caffeine, stating that the beverage can "Repress those vapours which the head invade." Also, Waller refers to tea as "The Muse's friend," which is obviously a reference to the ability of tea to enhance creativity in the drinker.

Edith Bynum, "Catherine of Braganza—England's First Tea Drinking Queen." *The Tea Caddy Newsletter*, November 2004. http://www.theteacaddy.com/Newsletter-November2004.htm.

and found the drink to be tasty and refreshing. Shennong, who is known as the father of Chinese medicine, is credited with discovering the medicinal value of tea.

The practice of drying and crushing tea leaves to produce fine flakes, resulting in a more potent cup of tea, began during China's Song Dynasty (A.D. 960–1279). It was also during this time that tea rituals were introduced into Chinese culture. Educated Chinese would read poetry, write calligraphy, paint, and discuss philosophy while enjoying tea.

Other Asian cultures also embraced tea consumption and adopted tea ceremonies. In Japan, for example, Buddhist monks introduced green tea during the twelfth century. This drink soon became very popular among the cultured people of Japan. Tea cultivation and consumption also spread to Vietnam, Korea, and other neighboring areas.

As European trade with Asia grew during the seventeenth and eighteenth centuries, tea became very popular in Europe, particularly among the wealthy classes. Catherine of Braganza, a Portuguese princess who became the wife of King Charles II, is generally credited with introducing tea to England around 1650. The drink became so popular in Great Britain that the British soon established tea plantations in their colony in India to cultivate the plants.

The Spread and Influence of Coffee

The Arabs were the first people to discover that coffee beans could be used to brew a refreshing hot drink. Arab traders brought coffee beans from Africa to Yemen, on the Arabian Peninsula, about a thousand years ago. The Arabs prepared a hot drink, which they called *qahwa*, by boiling green, uncooked coffee beans in water. During the late thirteenth century, the Arabs began roasting and grinding the coffee beans before adding them to boiling water; this improved the taste and made the drink even more popular.

Although for a time the Arabs of Yemen attempted to protect the secret of brewing coffee, by the fifteenth century

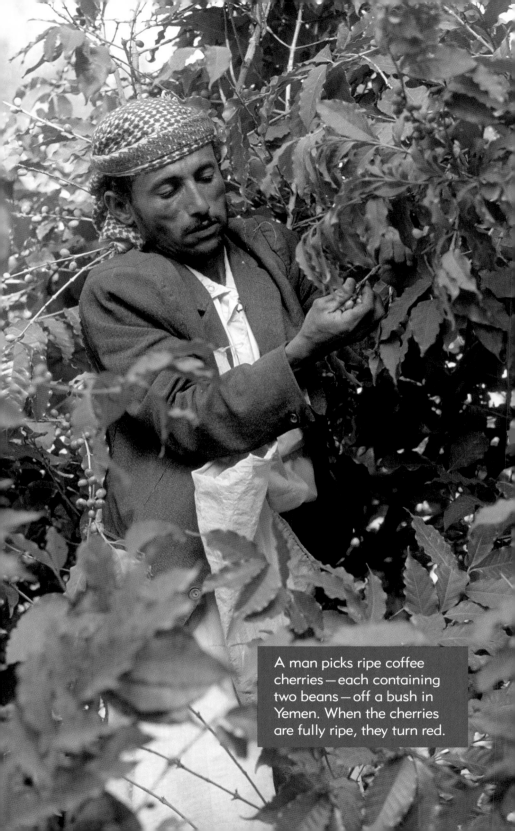

A man picks ripe coffee cherries—each containing two beans—off a bush in Yemen. When the cherries are fully ripe, they turn red.

coffee had become an accepted part of Arab culture as well as a popular beverage throughout the Turkish Ottoman Empire (which ruled the Arabian peninsula, as well as lands in northern Africa, eastern Europe, and central Asia). Gradually, Ottoman traders introduced coffee to neighboring cultures in eastern Europe.

At about the same time, the nations of western Europe were beginning to establish sea trade routes to Asia; coffee and tea were among the products the Dutch and Portuguese, among others, purchased from Arab or Asian merchants to sell in Europe. During the 1620s, Dutch traders started shipping coffee out of the Yemeni port of Mocha, establishing this Arabian city as the center of the Middle East's coffee trade. The Dutch traveler Pieter van den Broek wrote of coffee, "It is kind of black beans . . . of which they [the Arabs] make a black water and drink warm."[2]

This illustration shows people reading, writing, and conversing in an Istanbul coffee kiosk. Coffee became popular throughout the Ottoman Empire, and traders eventually brought the beverage to Europe.

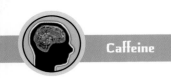

Cultivation of coffee plants eventually spread to areas outside of Africa and the Arabian peninsula. Dutch plantations on the Indonesian island of Java began growing coffee plants around 1699. (Today, both Mocha and Java are names for types of coffee.) The first coffee plantations in the Americas were established by the French on Martinique Island in 1720 and by the Portuguese in Brazil in 1727. As demand for coffee grew, the crop was imported to plantations in other European colonies in Central America, South America, and the Caribbean.

Caffeine in Europe

By the seventeenth century, consumption of coffee and tea had become common throughout Europe. The first coffeehouse in London opened in 1652; by 1675 there were some 3,000 coffeehouses in the city. These were popular places for the great intellectuals of the day. Writers like Daniel Defoe, Joseph Addison, and Richard Steele composed some of the most important English literature of the eighteenth century in London coffeehouses. Addison, author of the play *Cato* (a favorite of George Washington's) and copublisher of the influential newspaper *The Spectator*, believed the coffeehouse inspired his most original thoughts. He wrote, "I shall be ambitious to have it said of me that I brought philosophy out of the closets and libraries, schools and colleges, to dwell in clubs and assemblies, at tea-tables and coffeehouses."[3]

Coffeehouses could be found in other European capitals as well. In Paris, cafés were known as meeting places for writers, intellectuals, and philosophers, drawing such Enlightenment thinkers as Voltaire and Jean-Jacques Rousseau. (Voltaire was said to be fond of a brew that combined coffee and chocolate, giving the philosopher a double dose of caffeine.) When Benjamin Franklin served as American ambassador to France during the American Revolution, he often visited Paris coffeehouses to discuss the great ideas of the Enlightenment, particularly liberty and democracy.

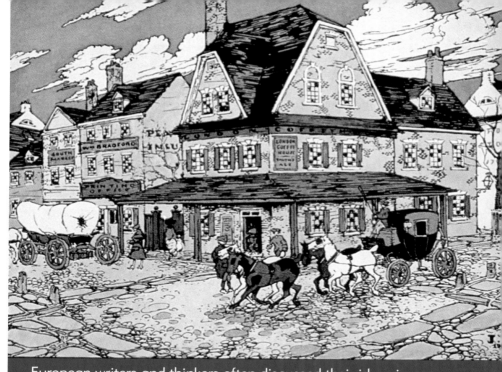

European writers and thinkers often discussed their ideas in coffeehouses like the one pictured here.

One dedicated and unabashed caffeine addict was the prolific French author Honoré de Balzac, who stayed up all night writing his many novels, essays, and stories (he published more than ninety during his lifetime). To stay awake, he drank coffee continuously. Balzac claimed the drink did more than just give him energy; he believed it cleared his mind and made him a better writer. In his 1839 essay "On Modern Stimulants," Balzac wrote,

> Coffee is a great power in my life; I have observed its effects on an epic scale. . . . Coffee sets the blood in motion and stimulates the muscles; it accelerates the digestive process, chases away sleep, and gives us the capacity to engage a little longer in the exercise of our intellects.[4]

Coffee and tea did more than stimulate the brains of European thinkers and artists. Some historians believe the arrival of caffeinated drinks in Europe may have contributed to healthier conditions in the crowded cities. The seventeenth and eighteenth centuries were a time when people did not understand that microscopic bacteria in food and water spread diseases. When water was boiled to make coffee or tea, the bacteria were destroyed; thus those who drank these beverages were less likely to catch infectious diseases like typhoid

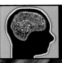 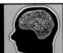

Charles II Bans Caffeine

British King Charles II worried that the lively conversation and edgy writing found in London's coffeehouses would lead to political unrest, so on December 29, 1675, the king issued a proclamation closing all English coffeehouses and prohibiting the sale of "Coffee, Chocolate, Sherbett, or Tea."

The king's proclamation stated that coffeehouses are "the great resort of Idle and disaffected persons . . . , have produced very evil and dangerous effects; as well for that many tradesmen and others, do herein mispend much of their time, which might and probably would be employed in and about there Lawful Calling and Affairs."

The king's proclamation was scheduled to go into effect on January 10, 1676. On January 8, Charles abruptly canceled the order, permitting the coffee shops to stay open. It is possible that the king feared his subjects would miss their coffee and tea so much they would rebel, but it is more likely he was reminded that the government collected taxes on coffee and tea sales, and that the kingdom would miss the revenue if the ban took effect.

Quoted in Bennett Alan Weinberg and Bonnie K. Bealer, *The World of Caffeine: The Science and Culture of the World's Most Popular Drug.* New York: Routledge, 2002, p. 159.

and dysentery. Others believe caffeine may have contributed to the success of the Industrial Revolution of the eighteenth and nineteenth centuries, by giving factory workers energy and helping them to work long hours. As T.R. Reid explained in an article for *National Geographic*:

> It is hardly a coincidence that coffee and tea caught on in Europe just as the first factories were ushering in the industrial revolution. The widespread use of caffeinated drinks—replacing the ubiquitous beer—facilitated the great transformation of human economic endeavor from the farm to the factory. Boiling water to make coffee or tea helped decrease the incidence of disease among workers in crowded cities. And the caffeine in their systems kept them from falling asleep over the machinery. In a sense, caffeine is the drug that made the modern world possible.[5]

By the early 1800s, some scientists had started looking for the reason coffee and tea were so popular. In 1819, German scientist Friedrich Ferdinand Runge isolated a stimulant in the coffee bean that he called "caffeine." In 1838, chemists discovered caffeine in tea.

The Rise of Caffeinated Soft Drinks

Once caffeine was isolated, it was only a matter of time before people would start to add it to other products. Among the first of these were carbonated drinks, which had their origin in the late eighteenth century. During the 1770s, an English chemist named Joseph Priestly developed a way to dissolve carbon dioxide gas in water. He promoted this carbonated water as a refreshing drink.

During the nineteenth century, as the temperance movement, which sought to ban consumption of alcohol, spread in the United States, various flavored carbonated drinks grew more popular. These became known as soft drinks (distinguished from "hard" drinks that contained alcohol). Among the most popular were such drinks as ginger ale and root beer.

These were produced in small quantities and sold locally. Neither ginger ale nor root beer contained caffeine. The first soft drink bottled commercially in the United States was Vernor's ginger ale, in 1866.

Twenty years later, an American pharmacist named John Styth Pemberton created what would become the world's most popular caffeinated soft drink: Coca-Cola. His formula for the drink included two natural stimulants: a small amount of cocaine, from the leaves of the coca plant, and caffeine, from kola nuts added to the drink for flavor.

In 1888, Pemberton sold the formula for Coca-Cola to another pharmacist, Asa Candler. The new owner advertised the drink as a patent medicine that would cure headaches, exhaustion, and other ailments. Eventually, Candler's Coca-Cola Company was forced to remove the cocaine from the drink's formula, but caffeine remained a key ingredient of the beverage. Candler changed his marketing strategy, advertising Coca-Cola as a refreshing drink, rather than as a medicine.

Other caffeinated soft drinks soon followed. During the 1890s, a pharmacist in North Carolina named Caleb Bradham developed a drink also flavored with kola nuts. Pepsi-Cola, as Bradham's drink was named in 1898, eventually became one of the most popular drinks in the world.

Caffeine on Trial

As caffeinated soft drinks like Coca-Cola and Pepsi grew in popularity, some people worried that they might cause dangerous health effects. The late 19th century and the early 20th century was a time of increased government regulation of the food and beverage industries. In 1906, at the urging of Dr. Harvey Washington Wiley, the head of the U.S. Bureau of Chemistry (the forerunner of the Food and Drug Administration), Congress passed the U.S. Pure Food and Drug Act. The new law was designed to put patent medicine companies out of business by making them list their ingredients on product labels. The regulations were too vigorous for

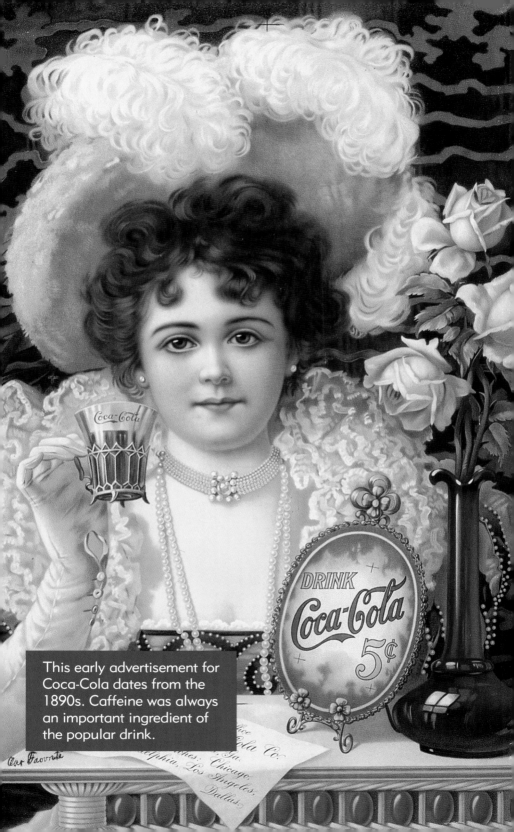

This early advertisement for Coca-Cola dates from the 1890s. Caffeine was always an important ingredient of the popular drink.

most elixir and tonic manufacturers, and many soon went out of business.

Next, Wiley turned his attention toward soft drink manufacturers, which he believed were making harmful products. Wiley was particularly concerned about the caffeine content of soft drinks; he felt this would harm the children who enjoyed the drinks. In 1909, Wiley ordered federal agents to seize a shipment of Coca-Cola just outside Chattanooga, Tennessee. Next, at Wiley's urging, the government filed a federal lawsuit against Coca-Cola, alleging that caffeine was a harmful ingredient of the company's product. The case went to trial in 1911.

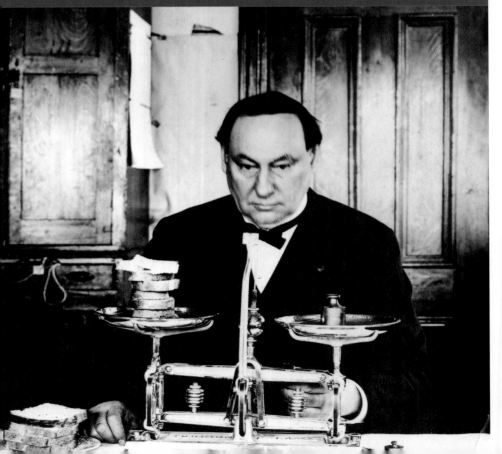

Dr. Harvey Washington Wiley failed in his effort to have caffeine-containing soft drinks removed from the market.

The testimony in *United States vs. Forty Barrels and Twenty Kegs of Coca-Cola* proved to be quite sensational. The lead witness for the prosecution was a streetcar conductor named Edwin H. Corry, who testified that Coca-Cola had caused him to hallucinate. Corry's physician, Dr. Sherman Clouting, testified, "He said he saw faces of people around him at night, that he heard distant music in his ears. He said he got very melancholy at times and had suicidal ideas, and when I asked him if he saw other visions, he said yes, he had seen the devil once or twice and the devil had touched him once."[6] Yet when Coca-Cola's lawyers specifically asked Clouting whether the caffeine content of their client's drink had caused Corry's paranoia, the doctor admitted that it had not. Corry, the doctor said, was probably already mentally ill before he started drinking Coca-Cola.

Support for Caffeine's Benefits

The judge hearing the case gave more weight to the testimony of Harry Hollingworth, a Columbia University psychology professor who, along with his wife and research assistant Leta, had been hired by Coca-Cola to test the effect of caffeine on human health. In a 150-page report, the Hollingworths wrote that a consumer would have to ingest more than 700 milligrams of caffeine in order to become sleep deprived. That was more than twenty times the dose of caffeine found in a glass of Coca-Cola. Rather than being dangerous, the Hollingworths' report found that in moderate dosages caffeine sharpened a person's reflexes.

The judge ruled in favor of Coca-Cola, finding that caffeine was not dangerous. In addition, because the caffeine came naturally from the kola nuts used to flavor the drink, the company could not be considered guilty of spiking its drink with the chemical, in his opinion. However, Coca-Cola was sensitive to the bad publicity generated by the trial, and company executives pledged not to feature children in Coca-Cola advertisements. It was a pledge they maintained until the 1980s.

Caffeine-Related Innovations

Over the past century, there have been many innovations related to caffeine. In 1901, a Japanese scientist named Sartori Kato developed a method for producing instant coffee. By the late 1930s, instant coffee was commercially available, allowing coffee drinkers in a hurry to simply drop a teaspoon or two of powdered and processed grounds into a cup of hot water. During World War II, American servicemen were issued packets of instant coffee in their mess kits.

Tea became easier to brew as well. In 1904, tea merchant Thomas Sullivan perfected the tea bag, taking what had been a relatively messy procedure (tea leaves had to be strained through a filter) and making it as easy as dropping a tiny paper sack into a cup of boiling water.

Chocolate consumption also became more widespread with the development of the candy bar in the late nineteenth century. Milton S. Hershey founded one of the most successful candy companies in 1900. Three years later, he built a plant to process chocolate bars near Harrisburg, Pennsylvania (the name of the town where the plant was constructed would eventually be changed to Hershey). The milk chocolate bars made at this plant proved to be very popular, and within a few years Hershey was the largest candy manufacturer in the country.

Another important change occurred in 1902, when the Barcolo Manufacturing Company of Buffalo, New York, introduced a new concept on its factory floor: the coffee break. Once in midmorning and once in midafternoon, production came to a stop as all employees were granted a fifteen-minute break to enjoy a cup of coffee. At Barcolo, an executive told a local newspaper,

> The employees felt like they needed a mid-morning and mid-afternoon break . . . and one of the employees volunteered to heat the coffee up on a kerosene-fueled hot plate. The employees paid for the coffee . . . and started taking, obviously with the approval of management,

about a 10- to 15-minute, mid-morning and mid-afternoon coffee break.[7]

The Barcolo executives probably were pleasantly surprised at the caffeinated workers' pace of production at the conclusion of their breaks, and soon other industries were offering their employees coffee breaks at work.

Of course, office workers are not the only people who start their days with caffeine. Many factory workers, tradespeople, bus drivers, housewives, teachers, and students routinely

A shipyard worker pauses for a cup of coffee, circa 1941. During the twentieth century the coffee break became widely accepted in American factories, offices, and other workplaces.

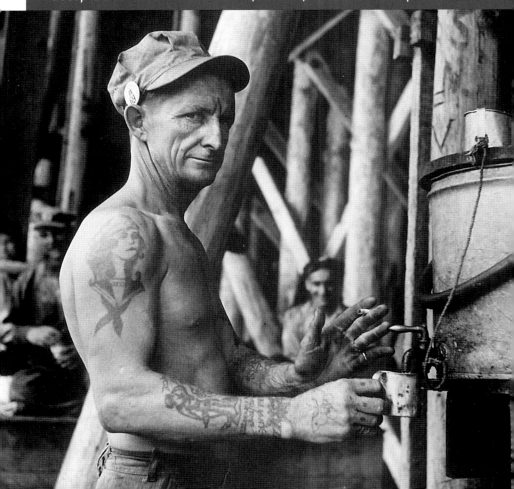

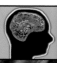
Caffeinated Water
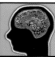

People who do not enjoy coffee, tea, or soft drinks but still want a caffeine jolt have an alternative: caffeinated water. There are now several brands of bottled water on the market that have been enhanced with caffeine.

Some people have used caffeinated water in an unexpected way—to make coffee. This gives the drink an extra caffeine kick. One connoisseur of coffee made with caffeinated water, was Omaha, Nebraska, radio talk show host Rocket Phillips. He told the *New York Times*, "We made our coffee with it. Everyone was buzzing around pretty good."

Barnaby J. Feder, "The Latest Mousetrap: Caffeine-Laced Spring Water," *New York Times*, May 6, 1996, p. A10.

consume coffee or other caffeinated drinks, believing that they are essential to getting their brains working.

In 1969, Stanford University School of Medicine researchers Avram Goldstein and Sophia Kaizer asked 239 housewives about what they liked about coffee. While a handful of respondents claimed the main reason they drank coffee was because they enjoyed the taste, the majority said they needed coffee to get going in the morning. Edward M. Brecher discussed this survey in his book *Licit and Illicit Drugs*, and noted:

A special subgroup of the morning coffee drinkers consisted of 25 housewives who drank coffee before breakfast. This group was particularly aware of the drug effect of the coffee; 80 percent reported that it "helps you wake up," 56 percent that it "gives you a lift," and 44 percent that it "stimulates you." In this group, moreover, 60 percent reported that they drink coffee in the morning because they "feel the need for it."[8]

Caffeine on the Cutting Edge

Coffee and other caffeinated drinks remain very popular among people of all ages. Anybody who doubts how much Americans enjoy caffeine need only look at the explosive growth of the gourmet coffee industry over the past quarter century. In 2005, for example, the Starbucks chain of coffee shops earned more than $5 billion in revenue.

In addition to strong, high-priced coffee, establishments like Starbucks offer cappuccinos, espressos, lattes, and other exotic drinks, many seasoned with spices and topped off with foamy clouds of cream. Frequenters of these coffee bars can enjoy their favorite beverages while music plays in the background, and can often surf the Internet using their laptops by

Today coffee shops like the one pictured here have become places where young people can log onto the Internet using wi-fi connections while enjoying a cup of coffee.

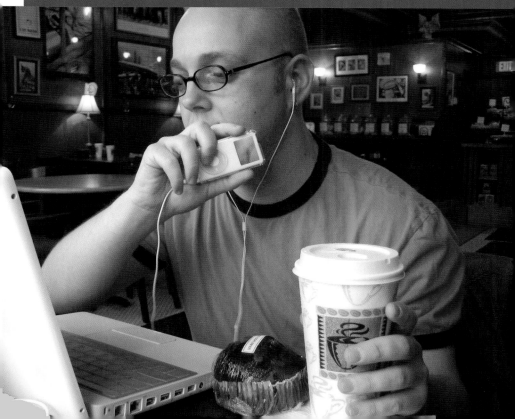

tapping into the store's wireless network. Today, there are more than 8,500 Starbucks locations in some thirty countries.

Author Bennett Alan Weinberg said he is not surprised that Starbucks grew first in the Seattle area—one of the nation's high-tech hubs. He explained,

> There isn't a computer company in the world that doesn't have Coke machines and coffee machines readily available; they supply it free to their people. Now this isn't just because coffee can help wake you up and, therefore, may help you to work a little longer; it aids in hand-eye coordination so you can key things in more accurately. Maybe more important, it also increases verbal fluency, it increases memory, it increases the ability to do calculations more accurately and it may stimulate creative thought, too. So the fact is [caffeine] has become the drug of the computer world.[9]

Other caffeinated beverages remain extremely popular among young workers and students. The Coca-Cola Company had $5.3 billion in worldwide sales during 2004, while Red Bull, one of the most popular energy drinks, sold 1.9 billion cans, generating about $2 billion in revenue, in 2004.

Minor and Temporary Health Effects

People who consume caffeine should understand how the drug affects the human brain and body. Caffeine provides definite benefits, such as increased alertness, but too much of the drug can make it hard for people to relax or fall asleep. For the most part, caffeine's effects on the brain and body are minor and temporary. However, there can be health risks when too much caffeine is consumed, such as elevated heartbeat and muscle aches. When physicians talk to their patients about what may be the right amount of caffeine for them, they invariably use one word: moderation.

Chapter 2

How Caffeine Impacts Human Health

Caffeine is a stimulant. It makes people alert, gives them energy, and helps make them active. Many people believe that if they do not start the day with a cup of coffee or tea, they are likely to be drowsy and unable to concentrate. Yale University pharmacology professor J. Murdoch Ritchie explains,

> Caffeine stimulates all portions of the [cerebral] cortex. Its main action is to produce a more rapid and clearer flow of thought, and to allay drowsiness and fatigue. After taking caffeine one is capable of a greater sustained intellectual effort and a more perfect association of ideas. . . . In addition, motor activity is increased; typists, for example, work faster and with fewer errors.[10]

Blocking Neurotransmitters

Like all drugs, caffeine affects neurotransmitters, the chemicals that deliver messages from brain cell to brain cell. Neurotransmitters affect how the brain and body function—they control emotions, coordination, and speech. Caffeine blocks the release of the neurotransmitter adenosine, which acts as

31

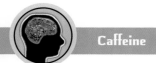
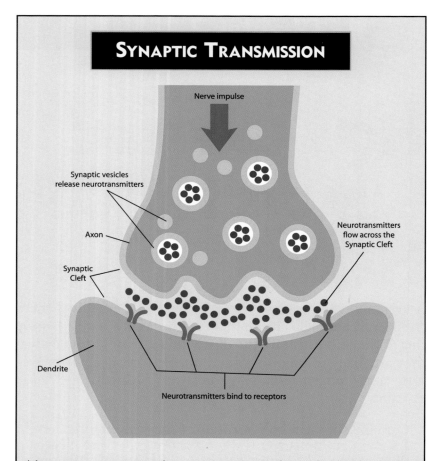

SYNAPTIC TRANSMISSION

Nerve impulse

Synaptic vesicles release neurotransmitters

Axon

Synaptic Cleft

Neurotransmitters flow across the Synaptic Cleft

Dendrite

Neurotransmitters bind to receptors

Neurons process and carry messages from the body to the brain and central nervous system. These messages, or impulses, must be transmitted across gaps between the neurons (synapses). This is accomplished with the help of chemicals called neurotransmitters, which are released from synaptic vesicles in the axon of a nerve cell. They carry the impulse across the synapse, and bind with receptors in the dendrite of an adjacent neuron. This allows the impulse to quickly move through the nervous system to the brain. Drugs like caffeine affect the way that neurotransmitters work, and this produces the drug's effect on a user's brain and body.

an inhibitor of the other neurotransmitters. When adenosine flows normally through the brain, it slows down the brain and body. This chemical helps people rest and sleep at night. But when adenosine is blocked, the brain and body become more alert and active, because the body responds by releasing another neurotransmitter, the hormone epinephrine (also called adrenaline). The effects of epinephrine include increased heart rate and blood pressure. It also causes some blood vessels to expand, resulting in greater blood flow to the muscles, and makes others contract, decreasing blood flow to the skin and inner organs.

Caffeine also increases the level of another neurotransmitter, dopamine, in the brain. This chemical is crucial to the function of certain areas of the brain, particularly those that control physical movements, memory, and attention. The release of dopamine also creates feelings of pleasure in the caffeine user. (Caffeine produces a more mild effect than some other drugs that also affect the release of dopamine, such as cocaine or amphetamines.)

Once caffeine is consumed, it takes about thirty minutes before the effects are felt. The effects reach their peak in about sixty minutes, then gradually wear off. Caffeine's most pronounced effects are usually dispelled after about three-and-a-half hours (if, that is, the person has not ingested more caffeine). Studies have shown, though, that caffeine remains in the blood for many hours after the initial rush has worn off and that the drug continues to exert a subtle, but nevertheless significant, effect on the body and brain.

Caffeine's Effect on Sleep

Caffeine is best known for its effect on sleep. Someone who consumes a cup of coffee near bedtime will probably not sleep well. In fact, some researchers believe that people who drink as little as two cups of coffee a day are likely to have their sleep cycles interrupted, even if they stop consuming caffeine several hours before they are ready for bed.

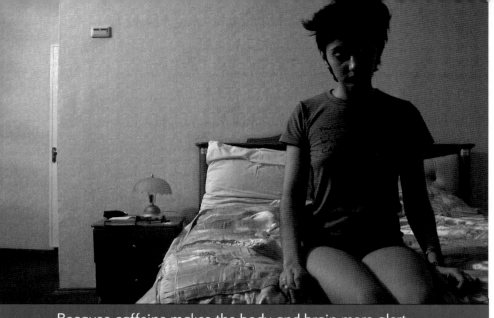

Because caffeine makes the body and brain more alert, sleeplessness can be a problem when the drug is consumed in the evening.

Most people who stop drinking coffee by midday can fall asleep quickly enough; the concern for sleep researchers relates to the depth and quality of their sleep. In his book *Caffeine Blues*, nutritionist Stephen Cherniske cited studies that demonstrate how regular caffeine use interrupts sleep, causing its consumers to wake often during the night. This frequent wakefulness means they are unable to remain for any length of time in the Stage Four sleep period—the times during the night in which people experience the deepest, most restful sleep. One study conducted in Zurich, Switzerland, showed that people who consumed two hundred milligrams of caffeine at seven o'clock in the morning—about the equivalent of two regular-strength cups of coffee—still had caffeine in their blood at eleven o'clock at night, even though they had taken no more caffeine after their morning doses. Even though such coffee drinkers may have no problem falling asleep, they may still wake up tired. Cherniske wrote,

> I don't think it is being overly cynical to suggest that this is precisely what the caffeine industry wants. After all, if you're groggy in the morning, you'll reach for

their product. . . . You fell asleep but never got to experience the depth of sleep that you need most. Is the problem widespread? Recent surveys suggest that 25 percent of U.S. adults have trouble falling asleep, 23 percent awaken frequently, 25 percent wake up too early, nearly half of all Americans are dissatisfied with the quality of their sleep, and one out of every ten is taking some medication to help them sleep.[11]

Young people who consume a lot of caffeine—usually in chocolate or soft drinks—often have difficulty falling asleep. A 2003 study examined the sleeping patterns of 191 seventh-, eighth-, and ninth-grade students. The young people involved in the study recorded caffeine use that ranged from zero to eight hundred milligrams a day, although most of the participants averaged about sixty-three milligrams a day. The study determined that teenagers who consumed the most

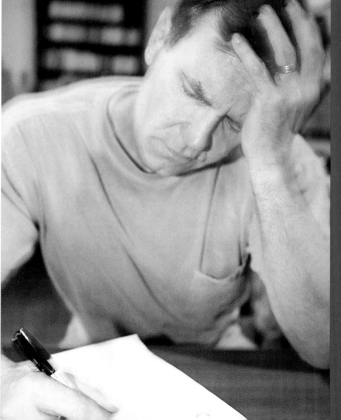

Too much caffeine can disrupt a person's sleep cycle. On awakening, the groggy person feels compelled to have another dose of the drug in order to activate his or her brain.

caffeine during the day had the most trouble sleeping at night, and were more likely to feel tired during the day. Researchers David Bright and Charles L. Pollack, who conducted the study, suggested a solution in their article about the study, which was published in the journal *Pediatrics*:

> The increasing availability of soft drink dispensing machines in schools is apparently welcomed by students and is profitable to school boards, but our findings suggest that it may be interfering with the nighttime sleep of teenagers. Pending additional studies that confirm or refute these findings, it may eventually become appropriate to limit the caffeine contents of soft drinks or restrict the types of beverages that are promoted to teenagers.[12]

A separate study released in 2004 concluded that many adolescents who consume large amounts of caffeine suffer from high blood pressure. The study found African-American teenagers were most affected, and at a higher risk for hypertension, a chronic condition caused by high blood pressure that can lead to a variety of health issues, including heart attack and stroke.

Dehydration Danger

Caffeine is a diuretic, which means it causes frequent urination. People who urinate frequently risk dehydration, which is a potentially dangerous condition caused by a lack of fluids in the body. What doctors find troubling is that when coffee drinkers dehydrate themselves, they often attempt to replace their lost fluids by drinking more coffee. As a result, all they are really doing is making themselves go to the bathroom even more; the diuretic effect of the caffeine means they lose even more fluids.

Although it is very rare for most coffee drinkers to suffer from the debilitating effects of dehydration—such as dizziness, fainting, low blood pressure, and blood in the urine and

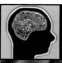

Caffeine and Jet Lag

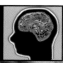

Long-distance travelers who cross many time zones often find themselves suffering from jet lag, a condition that occurs when the body adjusts to a change in the clock. For example, a traveler leaves New York City at six P.M., heads west to Los Angeles, and arrives there five hours later. To the traveler, it is 11 P.M.—time for bed—when he or she arrives. However, because the West Coast is three time zones behind New York, the traveler has arrived at eight P.M. according to clocks in Los Angeles. If the traveler decides to follow Los Angeles time, and does not go to bed for another three hours, the traveler's internal clock will be thrown off. Sometimes it takes days for the body to adjust to a change in time zones.

In 2005, researchers in France recommended that jet-lagged travelers consume large quantities of caffeine until their bodies adjust to their new time zones. They recommended a strong cup of coffee at breakfast, then an additional cup every two or three hours. The French study suggested that travelers should stop drinking coffee four to six hours before bedtime. In their book *The Caffeine Advantage*, authors Bennett Alan Weinberg and Bonnie K. Bealer added, "The actions of caffeine have been proven to increase attention span and vigilance, improve verbal fluency, and boost short-term memory. So in addition to helping reset your body clock, caffeine acts as a specific antidote that counteracts the most damaging impairments caused by jet lag and helps us to function normally even when we find ourselves in the grip of the condition."

Bennett Alan Weinberg and Bonnie K. Bealer, *The Caffeine Advantage*. New York: Free Press, 2002, p. 54.

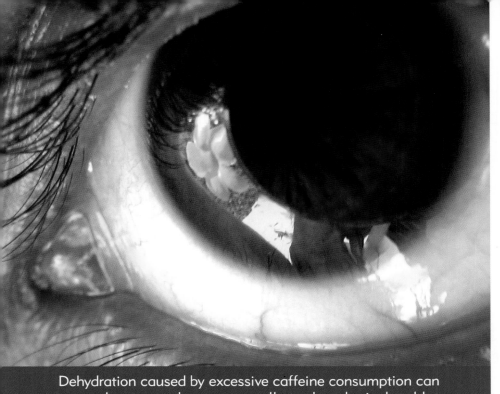

Dehydration caused by excessive caffeine consumption can cause damage to the eyes, as well as other physical problems.

stool—one place where caffeine's dehydrating effects can commonly show up is in the eyes. "I find it remarkable that so little attention has been paid to the role of caffeine in eye health," wrote Cherniske in *Caffeine Blues.* "Caffeine's diuretic effect can make your eyes so dry that wearing contact lenses is uncomfortable or impossible."[13]

The degree of dehydration that caffeine consumers suffer may also show up in their bowel movements. Dehydration reduces the water in the digestive tract, which causes constipation. On the other hand, when caffeine is consumed on an empty stomach it can cause diarrhea. If this occurs regularly over a period of time, the body adjusts to the caffeine intake and the diarrhea stops. However, if the person stops drinking coffee, tea, or soft drinks, they find themselves constipated until their body adjusts again. Therefore, caffeine has the distinction of being among the few drugs known to modern science that causes diarrhea and constipation.

Long-Term Health Effects

The short-term effects of caffeine, like sleeplessness and dehydration, are well known by scientists. In recent years, medical researchers have attempted to better understand how long-term caffeine use affects the human body. Some studies have uncovered disturbing trends. However, the research into the potential health risks of caffeine is ongoing, and to date there have been no reasons for the U.S. Food and Drug Administration to place controls on the caffeine content of foods and beverages.

One area being studied is whether there is a relationship between heavy caffeine use and heart failure. Some researchers have found that people who suffer heart attacks are often heavy coffee drinkers. However, heavy caffeine use on its own might not be a direct cause of heart attacks, because most of the people studied had other factors that increased their risk for heart disease, such as drinking alcohol or smoking cigarettes. High caffeine use could therefore be a symptom of an unhealthy lifestyle, and that lifestyle—rather than the caffeine use—may be increasing people's chances of heart attack.

Another area in which research is ongoing is the effect of caffeine on the human immune system. Some studies seem to indicate that heavy caffeine use can weaken the immune system, making caffeine consumers more susceptible to disease. However, as with the heart disease study, much more research must be done before this link can be proven.

Caffeine has been found to aggravate a condition known as tinnitus—a ringing of the inner ear. Recent research has shown that caffeine also can aggravate some muscle ailments, such as tennis elbow, neck pain, and carpal tunnel syndrome (a condition causing pain and weakness in the fingers and hands, suffered by some computer keyboard users and others engaged in repetitive hand motion). Caffeine also can cause heartburn and aggravate other stomach problems, such as ulcers.

Some people are allergic to caffeine and will develop unpleasant symptoms if they are exposed to the drug.

Consumers' Research cited one case of a fifty-three-year-old man who developed hives after consuming a caffeinated product; it also reported on the case of a fifty-year-old woman who lost her ability to walk and speak clearly. Her ailment was traced to an allergic reaction to coffee.

Caffeine-Related Deaths Rare

It is possible for a person to die from a caffeine overdose, but such cases are very rare. For starters, it takes an enormous amount of caffeine—about the equivalent of one hundred cups of coffee—to cause the condition known as "caffeine intoxication." Consuming that much caffeine can cause muscle spasms, shock, convulsions, vomiting, and a racing heart.

Just as accidental deaths caused by caffeine are extremely unlikely, suicides due to caffeine overdose are rare as well, even though caffeine pills are readily available. In *The World of Caffeine*, authors Weinberg and Bealer explain that caffeine is rarely employed as a suicide drug because most people simply do not regard caffeine as a deadly substance. "Caffeine may be used to commit suicide so infrequently partially because few people know if it could kill them or how much it would take to kill them,"[14] they wrote.

Still, an occasional story about a caffeine-related death appears in the news. In November 1998, a twenty-year-old college student named Jason Allen died in Morehead City, North Carolina, after swallowing dozens of caffeine pills on a dare. Police estimated that he ingested about eighteen grams of caffeine, or the equivalent of about 250 cups of coffee. And in November 2004, a forty-year-old woman named Ruth Ann Smith died soon after arriving at a hospital in Santa Fe, New Mexico. An autopsy revealed that she had consumed a massive dose of caffeine shortly before her death. It was suspected that she swallowed a whole bottle of an over-the-counter painkiller that contains caffeine. Tim Stepetic, a spokesman for the Santa Fe Office of the Medical Investigator, told the *Albuquerque Journal* that the caffeine level in

Smith's body was "extremely, extremely high, maybe three times the lethal limit for caffeine in the body."[15] Smith's death was ruled a suicide by caffeine overdose.

Caffeine and Pregnancy

In recent years, medical research has focused on the effect of caffeine on children and adolescents. But so far, the only action the Food and Drug Administration has taken regarding caffeine use is to issue a warning to pregnant women that heavy consumption of caffeine could cause miscarriages. It is believed that some 75 percent of pregnant women in the United States consume caffeine and that about 30 percent consume large amounts. In 1996, Yale University School of Medicine studied the consumption of caffeinated beverages by women in their first month of pregnancy. The researchers concluded that heavy caffeine intake is a direct cause of miscarriage.

The Yale University study also reported that heavy caffeine consumption also contributes to other factors that may cause a difficult pregnancy—such as lack of sleep and stress by the mother. A second study cited by *Consumers' Research* magazine reported that for each one hundred milligrams ingested daily by a pregnant woman, the risk of miscarriage increases by 22 percent.

Doctors advise pregnant women to limit or eliminate their caffeine intake, because the drug is believed to increase the risk of miscarriage.

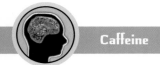

Research shows that when a pregnant woman drinks a cup of coffee or a caffeinated soft drink, the caffeine enters the body of the fetus. However, the fetus's undeveloped liver does not yet have the ability to eliminate the drug from the body, so caffeine stays in the fetus longer than it would in an adult. This can lead to physical problems.

For example, one study conducted in New Zealand focused on mothers who consumed caffeine daily during their pregnancies. It concluded that babies with high concentrations of caffeine in their bodies may be born with respiratory problems, which may lead to Sudden Infant Death Syndrome (SIDS). This is a syndrome which causes the tragic death of otherwise healthy babies in their cribs or playpens for no apparent reason. The New Zealand study found that in 393 of 1,592 cases of SIDS (25 percent), mothers of babies who

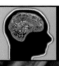 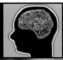

Caffeine Guidelines for Kids

Although the U.S. government has no guidelines on caffeine consumption by young children, the Canadian government has made recommendations to parents. For children between the ages of four and six, the Canadian government recommends that caffeine consumption be limited to no more than forty-five milligrams a day—about the equivalent of a twelve-ounce can of soda. For children between the ages of seven and nine, the Canadian government recommends no more than sixty-three milligrams of caffeine a day, or about one-and-a-half servings of soda. For children between the ages of ten and twelve, the recommendation is for no more than eighty-five milligrams—not quite two cans of soda.

died consumed at least four hundred milligrams of caffeine a day during their pregnancies.

University of California toxicologist Brenda Ezkanazy told a reporter for National Public Radio, "Given all of this information and the fact that we can control our exposure to caffeine, it's probably in the best interest of the fetus that we limit our intake as much as possible."[16]

Caffeine's Impact on Young Children

Young children also suffer negative effects from consuming caffeine. Preschoolers who drink caffeinated beverages or eat chocolate candy often have behavioral problems. They can also have trouble concentrating. As with the fetus, this is because children's bodies can not remove the caffeine from their systems as quickly as an adult. When a child who is perhaps a third or a quarter of the body weight of an adult consumes the same quantity of caffeinated soda, the effect of the drug is multiplied.

One study on caffeine's effect on young children was performed at the University of Minnesota. Child psychiatrists gave several children ages eight through twelve two or three cans of caffeinated drinks a day for thirteen days, then substituted caffeine-free drinks without telling them. A day after switching the children to caffeine-free drinks, the psychiatrists administered tests to the children and concluded that the test subjects experienced decreased attention spans as well as headaches and feelings of tiredness.

Pediatricians and childrens' health experts have other concerns about caffeinated drinks that are not directly related to their caffeine levels. For example, when children drink soda, they are likely to drink less milk, which means they will not receive the calcium they need to build strong bones. At the same time, because most soft drinks are heavily sweetened, children risk obesity and tooth decay. These effects make most nutritionists concerned about the amount of caffeinated soft drinks that young children consume.

The Positive Benefits of Caffeine

Researchers have discovered that caffeine has many positive effects on human health. For example, it has been known for years that caffeine can be an effective analgesic, particularly for headache sufferers. In fact, a remedy for a migraine headache has always been a strong cup of black coffee. Today, therefore, many over-the-counter headache remedies include caffeine, a fact that is stated clearly on these pills' labels. Such pills work because one of the functions of the neurotransmitter adenosine is to carry certain pain signals in the brain. When caffeine blocks the adenosine, it also prevents pain signals from reaching the brain and thus deadens headache pain.

Caffeine can help overweight and obese people lose weight by increasing their metabolism. Studies have found that caffeine increases the basal metabolic rate—the rate at which the body burns energy while at rest—by as much as 25 percent. This makes the body more efficient at burning calories, and helps a person who is dieting to shed pounds. Moreover, caffeine helps to suppress the appetite, making a person less likely to snack between meals.

Caffeine's diuretic effect can also have positive benefits. As one study found, coffee drinkers suffer fewer kidney stones—painful accumulations of waste that solidify in the kidneys and occasionally require surgery to remove.

A Harvard University study found that caffeine speeds the delivery of insulin to human tissue. Insulin is a protein that helps the body convert sugar into energy. A person who does not produce enough insulin could develop diabetes, a potentially debilitating disease which can cause cardiovascular disease, chronic renal failure, retinal damage that can lead to blindness, and other significant health problems. But the Harvard study found that coffee drinkers are less likely to develop diabetes, probably because of the way caffeine enhances the performance of insulin in the body.

Studies have also indicated that caffeine may be beneficial in helping to prevent other serious diseases, including colon

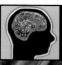
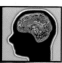
U.S. soldiers often find it impossible to stop for a coffee break. So to get their caffeine jolt, some soldiers stuff a wad of instant coffee between their lower lip and bottom gum, similar to how chewing tobacco is used. "The granules form a gel-like substance and offer a noticeable

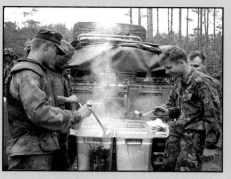

Marines break from training to make instant coffee and tea using hot water.

caffeine kick," reported the military newspaper *Stars and Stripes*. "The bitter goo would never be mistaken for a gourmet brew, but it does the trick."

The military has studied the effect of caffeine on soldiers. Commando trainees, for example, have to go without sleep for long periods, while performing intense physical activities and enduring psychological stress. In one study, after three days of such training the recruits were given caffeine. When tested, the soldiers who had consumed the most caffeine recorded the highest scores. Dr. Harris R. Lierberman, a U.S. Army research psychologist, said, "This study demonstrated that even in the most adverse operational circumstances, moderate doses of caffeine had unequivocal, beneficial effects on cognitive performance."

Steve Mraz, "Reporter's Notebook: Trick for a Caffeine Jolt Is far from Gourmet, But It'll Do," *Stars and Stripes*, October 4, 2005. www.estripes.com/article.asp?section=104&article=31191&archive=true.

National Coffee Association, "Caffeine Helps Keep Soldiers Vigilant and on Task," October 21, 2004. http://coffeescience.org/media/military.

cancer and Parkinson's disease. However, the research remains incomplete, and more study is needed to determine the degree to which caffeine can affect these diseases.

Safe in Moderation

All researchers agree that moderate use of caffeine is not harmful to health. Over the years, the drug has stood up to hundreds of tests, and they have all concluded that moderate use of caffeine will not shorten people's lives or lead to debilitating long-term conditions. Even pregnant women can enjoy an occasional cup of coffee without worrying about the impact of caffeine on their unborn babies. As author Stephen Braun wrote in his 1996 book *Buzz: The Science and Lore of Alcohol and Caffeine*, "The effects of caffeine on such things as breast cancer, bone loss, pancreatic cancer, colon cancer, heart disease, liver disease, kidney disease, and mental dysfunction have been examined in . . . detail and, to date, no clear evidence has been found linking moderate consumption of caffeine . . . with these or any other health disorder."[17]

Nevertheless, many heavy coffee drinkers who have decided they have had enough of sleepless nights and frequent trips to the bathroom decide to give up caffeine once and for all. They soon learn, though, that caffeine can be a highly addictive drug. Although it is certainly possible for them to kick their habits and live without their morning jolts of caffeine, they are likely to suffer many symptoms of withdrawal and to endure several bad days as their bodies adjust to a caffeine-free lifestyle.

Chapter 3

ADDICTED TO CAFFEINE

Researchers concluded more than a century ago that caffeine can create a physical addiction when overused. Heavy users who try to do without caffeine may feel physically or mentally incapable of functioning properly. Additionally, if they elect to stop ingesting caffeine completely, they may find themselves experiencing the physical symptoms of caffeine withdrawal. In an article in the January 1, 1998, edition of *Current Health 2,* Judy Monroe wrote, "Caffeine use creates both dependence and tolerance. . . . When you drink coffee, tea, or caffeine-laced soft drinks regularly, caffeine dependency can occur within a few days to a couple of weeks."[18]

Building a Tolerance
Heavy coffee drinkers often go to great extremes to satisfy their cravings for caffeine. In 2005, Michael Polino of Eggertsville, New York, told *Buffalo News* staff writer Anne Neville that he makes a pot of coffee every morning with enough water to brew eight cups—but he puts twelve scoops of ground coffee in the pot, meaning his brew is particularly strong. Polino told Neville, "My brother Dave says he drinks

coffee all day long, but I've had his coffee, and it's like drinking colored water! It's real weak."[19] In addition to drinking his own coffee throughout the day, Polino said he usually stops at a favorite coffee shop for a twenty-ounce cup of gourmet brew.

While interviewing self-described "coffee addicts" for a newspaper story, Neville spoke with Joe Koessler, owner of the Spot Coffee restaurant in Buffalo. He said that his restaurant's specialty is a double-strength shot of espresso—a particularly strong and bitter-tasting Italian coffee that contains as much caffeine in a two-ounce serving as a customer would find in an eight-ounce cup of regular coffee. Koessler said he has seen customers order four double-strength espresso shots. Barista Jenn Mayberry, a Spot Coffee employee, said that many caffeine addicts ask for what she called a "red eye"—a double-strength shot of espresso poured into a regular cup of coffee. "There was a guy who gets a red eye with

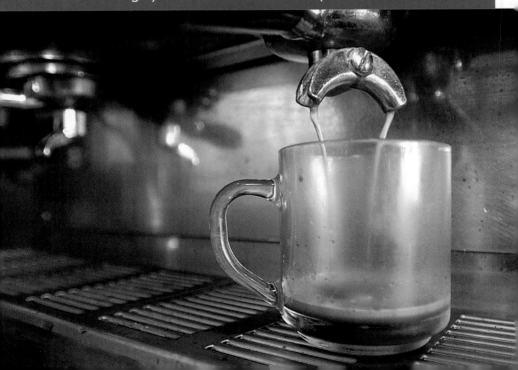

Some people become so dependent on a caffeine jolt that they seek out highly caffeinated drinks like espresso.

four (extra) double shots of espresso," Mayberry told Neville. "He came in every day, too."[20]

As addictions go, dependency on caffeine is relatively minor. However, caffeine does tend to take over some peoples' lives. In his book *Uncommon Grounds*, Mark Pendergrast interviewed a New York restaurant owner named Joe McBratney, who admitted to drinking the equivalent of fifty cups of coffee a day. Throughout the day, McBratney constantly fills and drains a coffee cup the size of a soup bowl. "I feel like a changed person after my first cup every morning," McBratney told Pendergrast. "I feel great."[21] Pendergrast believes McBratney has built up a caffeine tolerance, and that it requires larger and larger doses for him to achieve the buzz he craves.

Connoisseurs of soft drinks can also build up tolerances to caffeine. Judy Monroe interviewed teenager John Grabrick of Little Canada, Minnesota, who admitted that he consumes nearly 365 milligrams of caffeine each day. "As soon as I wake up in the morning, I head to the refrigerator, and pop open a can of cola. That's my breakfast. Each can gives me 140 calories and a great caffeine lift," he told Monroe. "I don't like coffee or tea. But I like caffeine's jolt, so I started drinking Coke. Now I go through eight 12-ounce cans each day. This 24-pack will last me three days."[22] As with McBratney, Grabrick has built up such a caffeine tolerance that now it takes large quantities of the drug to provide the stimulation he seeks.

Withdrawal Symptoms

McBratney, Grabrick, and other caffeine addicts face an unpleasant crash if they ever decide to quit using the drug. Those who stop using caffeine suddenly can expect sleepiness, lapses in concentration, decreased motivation, and irritability. Some caffeine addicts have also reported flulike symptoms, such as a runny nose, muscle aches, stiffness, hot and cold spells, nausea, vomiting, and blurred vision. The withdrawal symptoms typically begin within twelve hours of giving up caffeine and can last for as long as a week.

Some former caffeine users have even reported symptoms of depression—a mental illness in which sufferers may experience decreased appetite, difficulty concentrating, and, in some cases, an inability to get out of bed in the morning. These symptoms are probably caused by the return of adenosine to the user's brain and body. Adenosine helps the body relax, and when the body has been living on reduced levels of adenosine for an extended period (as is the case with heavy caffeine users), a sudden return of the neurotransmitter may result in the body becoming overrelaxed.

Painful Headaches

By far, the most common symptom of caffeine withdrawal is a splitting headache. Caffeine is known to constrict certain blood vessels, including some in the brain. Without the influence of caffeine, the blood vessels open wide to their normal size. The sudden rush of blood to the brain results in a nasty headache. The headaches can last as long as four days and in some cases longer, but they will go away once the body has adjusted. Bennett Alan Weinberg and Bonnie K. Bealer explain in their book, *The World of Caffeine: The Science and Culture of the World's Most Popular Drug*:

> Typically it is a generalized throbbing headache that can, in extreme cases, be accompanied by flulike symptoms such as nausea and vomiting. The caffeine withdrawal headache is worsened with physical exercise and, not surprisingly, is relieved by caffeine. The withdrawal headaches usually abate within two to four days, although some subjects continue reporting sporadic headaches for ten days or more after cessation of caffeine use.[23]

The headaches of caffeine withdrawal are not limited to coffee lovers. Pendergrast interviewed Cathy Rossiter, a

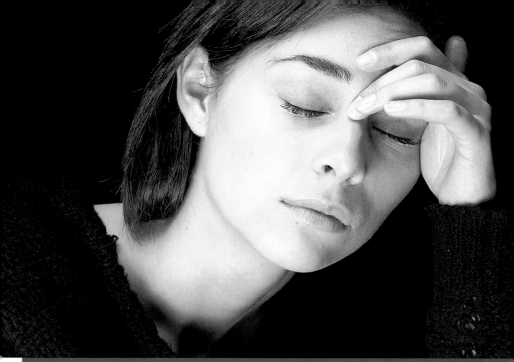

Strong headaches are a common symptom of caffeine withdrawal.

Mountain Dew drinker who struggled with headaches when she stopped ingesting the beverage. (Rossiter's addiction was so intense that she admitted to standing in a supermarket line, chugging down the beverage while in labor with her second child.) Rossiter took part in a Johns Hopkins Medical Center study of caffeine withdrawal symptoms. Just two days after she decided to stop drinking Mountain Dew, Rossiter told Pendergrast that she suffered from a terrible headache. "It felt like a migraine, just right behind your eyes. It was like someone had a little knife digging out your brains."[24] After just a few days in the study, Rossiter had enough of the Johns Hopkins test—she went back to drinking Mountain Dew.

John Grabrick told Judy Monroe that to prepare for knee surgery, he was told by his doctor not to eat or drink anything after nine o'clock the night before the operation. "When I woke up Wednesday morning, I had a huge headache and felt irritable," he said. "They wheeled me into surgery and gave me anesthesia to knock me out. When I woke up after the operation with a severe headache, the first words I mumbled to my mom were, 'Get me a Coke.'"[25]

The instructions given to Grabrick before surgery and his reaction as he emerged from the anesthesia after surgery are common. In fact, anesthesiologists typically prohibit patients from eating or drinking anything for eight or twelve hours prior to their surgeries because patients may vomit if they have adverse reactions to the pain-deadening medications. For a long time, recovery room nurses wondered why patients waking up from anesthesia complained about headaches. Initially, they thought it might be some kind of reaction to the anesthesia. It was eventually determined that because the patients had not ingested their regular caffeinated beverages, they were experiencing caffeine withdrawal headaches. In recent years, some physicians have agreed to administer caffeine intravenously to patients during the sur-

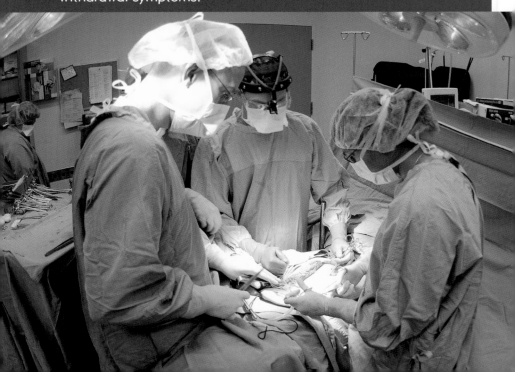

Doctors have found that after heavy caffeine users undergo prolonged surgical procedures, they sometimes suffer withdrawal symptoms.

gical procedures to help them avoid the headaches and other withdrawal symptoms as they recover from their operations.

Symptoms Vary in Strength

In general, the bigger the caffeine habit, the more acute the withdrawal symptoms can be. However, research has shown that withdrawal symptoms can occur even among those who drink just a cup of coffee or a couple of sodas each day. Weinberg and Bealer described this in *The Caffeine Advantage*:

> The seriousness of the physical and mental discomforts we experience when we suddenly stop using caffeine varies from person to person, depending on genetic constitution and the level of caffeine use. In general, the more caffeine you are taking, the stronger will be your physical dependence and the worse your withdrawal symptoms if you suddenly stop using caffeine. Levels as low as 100 mg a day have been found to support a physical dependence. That means that if you are drinking as little as one cup of coffee a day, you might feel slightly uncomfortable if you quit drinking coffee abruptly and cut out all other sources of caffeine as well.[26]

Men seem to have fewer caffeine withdrawal symptoms than women. This may be because men usually weigh more than women and, therefore, are more able than women to metabolize the caffeine. Stanley Segall, a professor of nutrition and food science at Drexel University in Philadelphia, told *Real Simple* magazine in 2004, "Men seem to clear caffeine from their systems faster than women do, just as they process alcohol faster."[27]

Psychological Dependence

While caffeine has been shown to cause physical dependence in some heavy users, many mental health experts believe the drug may also create a psychological dependence. In other words, some coffee drinkers believe they absolutely have to have a cup of coffee to get themselves going in the morning,

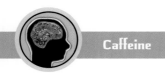

although physically they do not need the caffeine. People who have a psychological dependence on caffeine are said to suffer from "caffeinism."

In *The Caffeine Advantage*, Weinberg and Bealer explained that the typical person with a psychological dependence on caffeine will continue consuming the drug even after adverse effects related to their caffeine consumption become apparent. For example, they wrote, it is not unusual for a person who is psychologically dependent on caffeine to consume a cup of coffee late at night, even though he or she is aware that it will cause sleeping problems. The person believes so deeply that he or she needs the caffeine that he or she must consume it despite the consequences. People with a psychological dependence on caffeine also seek to constantly increase the strength of their caffeine jolt.

"This syndrome is uncommon, but, when it occurs, it is a clear sign that the person afflicted should markedly reduce or even eliminate caffeine intake, and seek professional counseling if necessary," wrote Weinberg and Bealer. "As Dr. Roland R. Griffiths, professor of psychiatry and behavioral pharmacology at Johns Hopkins University School of Medicine, one of the world's leading caffeine researchers, wrote to us, 'Use caffeine; don't let caffeine use you.'"[28]

Cutting Down Gradually

When heavy coffee drinkers decide to reduce or eliminate their caffeine intake, some may have a last binge, drinking large amounts of their favorite beverage. However, this is the wrong way to quit caffeine. Weinberg and Bealer explained in *The World of Caffeine*, "Several studies have found that both the likelihood of caffeine withdrawal and its severity increase as the daily dose attained before cessation is increased."[29] Therefore, it is not a good idea to drink a half dozen cups of coffee on the last day before quitting caffeine—the headache and other symptoms on the day after will be that much stronger.

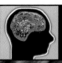 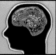

The Finns Drink the Most Coffee

Americans love their coffee—according to statistics compiled in 2003 by the International Coffee Organization, annually Americans consume what amounts to 280 cups of coffee per person. However, that rate of consumption ranks Americans in just fourteenth place among the world's coffee drinkers.

The biggest coffee consumers are the Finns, whose annual consumption is a robust 740 cups per person. (That equates to roughly twenty-eight pounds of coffee grounds per person.) In fact, citizens of the Scandinavian countries take four of the five top rankings for coffee drinking. After the Finns, Norwegians and Belgians tied for second place with an annual average of 634 cups. Danes came in fourth at 535 cups, and Swedes finished fifth at 525 cups.

Doctors advise caffeine users to cut down gradually. They suggest coffee drinkers start alternating cups of decaffeinated coffee with regular coffee over a period of several weeks, gradually replacing the real coffee with the decaf until, finally, they are consuming decaf only. Soft drink lovers can gradually switch to decaffeinated soft drinks, water, or fruit juices—although they should carefully check out the juices before they consume them because some fruit-flavored "high energy" drinks also contain caffeine.

In Baltimore, Johns Hopkins Medical Center has established a caffeine addiction clinic to help wean heavy caffeine users off the drug. One patient at the clinic, Lois Smith, told the CBS News Early Show in 2005 that at the peak of her caffeine addiction, she consumed twelve cups of coffee a day.

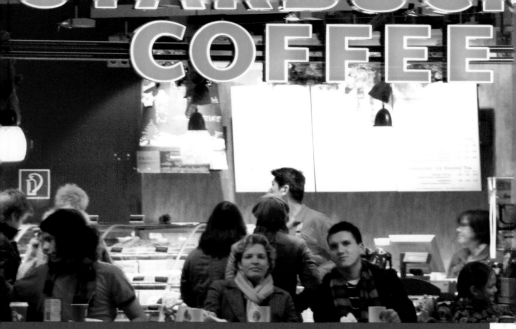

People who are psychologically addicted to caffeine may feel they need their favorite beverage — even at night, when they know it will interfere with their sleep.

"I'd wake up and my first thought was, 'Get to Starbucks and get a cup of coffee' so I could take it to work," she said. "There were times when my husband and I would go out to dinner after work and I would pick a restaurant because I knew that there was a Starbucks on the route."[30]

After Smith enrolled in the clinic, she was instructed to cut down on her caffeine by 25 percent for her first week. In the second week, she was instructed to reduce her caffeine consumption by 50 percent. Over the subsequent four weeks, she continued to gradually decrease her caffeine consumption. After six weeks, she was virtually caffeine free. "Now I wake up, I'm more rested, I'm more alert,"[31] she told CBS News.

However, just as recovered alcoholics and former smokers must constantly resist temptation, former caffeine addicts also must always be on guard. Although decaffeinated coffees and caffeine-free beverages are often available, Smith concedes that it takes willpower to sit down in a Starbucks and order a decaf. "Every once in awhile I'm a little shaky," she said.

"What I try to do is, before I come in, I make up my mind that I'm not gonna get a caffeinated beverage."[32]

Coffee, Cigarettes, and Addiction

Many people enjoy a cup of coffee and a cigarette together, and it is estimated that some 86 percent of smokers are also coffee drinkers. However, the link between the two is not just social. Scientists have found that caffeine has a special interaction with nicotine, the active ingredient in cigarettes. Nicotine speeds up the delivery of caffeine to the brain, heart, and other organs, making the caffeine rush more intense. The caffeine is also depleted faster in the body of a smoker. This means smokers need more caffeine to achieve the caffeine jolt. It also means the caffeine craving may return quicker in smokers than in nonsmokers.

Researchers are not sure why coffee drinking often goes hand in hand with smoking, but they do know that people

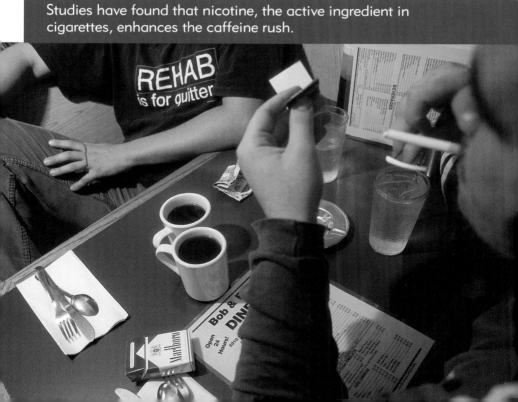

Studies have found that nicotine, the active ingredient in cigarettes, enhances the caffeine rush.

who drink coffee and smoke usually started using cigarettes after they had already established their caffeine habits. In her book *Dying to Quit: Why We Smoke and How We Stop*, author Janet Brigham wrote, "The relationship between caffeine use and nicotine consumption is probably at least partially behavioral. Coffee consumption and cigarette smoking are so frequently done together that either can serve as a cue that triggers the other, but smoking most often follows coffee consumption, not vice versa."[33]

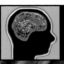 **Caffeine and Alcohol**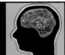

There is a common belief that drinking coffee will make an intoxicated person sober. However, scientists have found there is little truth to that belief. In two different studies, volunteers first drank alcohol to the point of intoxication, then consumed two cups of coffee. The coffee failed to sober up the volunteers — in fact, some of the volunteers who drank alcohol and coffee scored worse on performance tests than the volunteers who consumed alcohol only. Dr. Robert Forney of Indiana University reported, "In no instance did caffeine counteract the alcohol — and in many cases it made it worse."

There is no caffeinated drink a person can ingest that will enable their body to process alcohol faster. Alcohol will remain in the bloodstream for several hours, until it is naturally eliminated through the cleansing action performed by the liver.

Quoted in Frances Sheridan Goulart, *The Caffeine Book: A User's and Abuser's Guide.* New York: Dodd, Mead & Co., 1984, p. 33.

Cigarette smoking is a far riskier habit than consuming caffeine. The tar and nicotine content of cigarettes is directly linked to many serious and potentially fatal diseases, such as cancer, emphysema, stroke, and heart disease. Nicotine is much more physically and psychologically addictive than caffeine; most smokers face a difficult and lengthy trial when they try to quit smoking.

In *The World of Caffeine*, Weinberg and Bealer said it is often too much to ask a cross-addicted caffeine and nicotine user to give up both coffee and cigarettes simultaneously. Instead, they recommend that caffeine and nicotine users to at least cut down on coffee before they try to give up smoking.

Once a smoker gives up cigarettes, the nicotine will no longer enhance delivery of the caffeine. Therefore, the caffeine will not be burned as quickly, and it will remain in the body longer. "To put it simply," Weinberg and Bealer wrote, "if a heavy smoker is used to drinking four cups of strong coffee to wake up, he might find that, after discontinuing his cigarette habit, two cups will accomplish the same purpose."[34] But unless the coffee drinker realizes this fact and cuts down on coffee before giving up cigarettes, he or she may continue drinking four cups of coffee after quitting smoking—thereby becoming all the more addicted to caffeine.

Caffeine Helps Enhance Performance

Some people routinely consume large doses of caffeine and live very ordinary lives. Only when such people stop consuming caffeine do they experience withdrawal symptoms that can be unpleasant and painful, although only temporary. Still, the amount of caffeine a coffee lover consumes in a double-strength espresso is negligible when compared with the amounts some professional athletes consume. These athletes take in hundreds and even thousands of milligrams of caffeine for the energy lift they feel they need to compete. However, many people feel using caffeine to gain a competitive advantage is cheating.

Chapter 4

CAFFEINE AND SPORTS

When athletes take huge doses of caffeine, the drug can enable them to tap into enormous energy reserves and gain a competitive edge. However, many people are concerned about the caffeine habits of some top athletes. Doctors warn that supplements containing caffeine can be hazardous and even fatal. At the same time, most administrators of athletic organizations agree that any type of artificial boost that enhances performance borders on cheating and therefore should be banned from competition. They believe that there is little difference between caffeine and other performance-enhancing drugs, such as anabolic steroids, and wonder whether teaching young athletes to enhance their performance with drugs is wise.

How Caffeine Helps Athletes

In 1989, a *Sports Illustrated* reporter wrote about the weightlifting regimen of behemoth offensive tackle Tony Mandarich, a first-round draft choice of the Green Bay Packers. Before lifting weights, Mandarich, who is six feet six inches tall and weighs 315 pounds, consumed a sixteen-

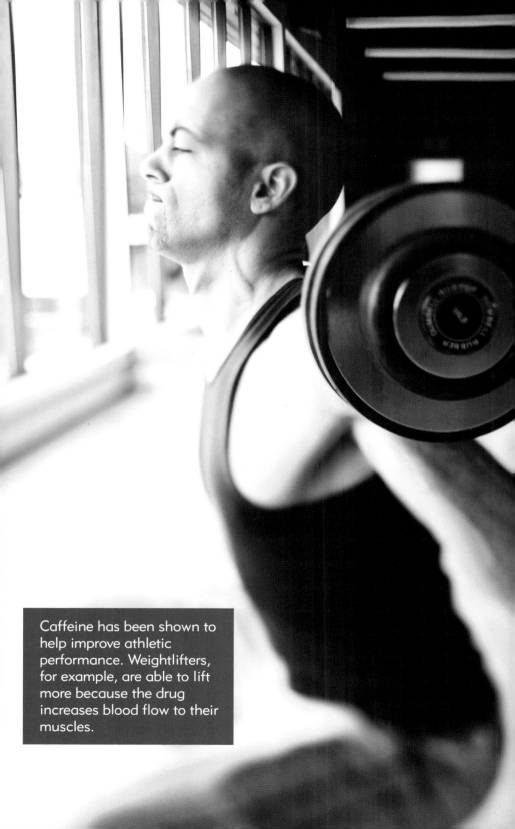

Caffeine has been shown to help improve athletic performance. Weightlifters, for example, are able to lift more because the drug increases blood flow to their muscles.

ounce bottle of highly caffeinated "Super Tea," thirty-two ounces of coffee, and a two hundred-milligram tablet of Vivarin. With all that caffeine working in his body, Mandarich started hoisting hundreds of pounds of weights. "If you're not going to be intense," remarked Mandarich to *Sports Illustrated* writer Rick Telander, "why come in?"[35]

By increasing blood flow to the muscles, the drug does help weightlifters, wrestlers, and other athletes who rely on their muscles to feel stronger. However, other athletes benefit from caffeine consumption as well. Caffeine has been shown to help long-distance runners, bicycle riders, and

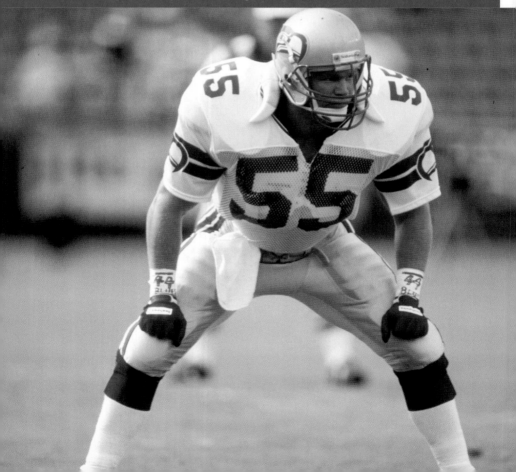

Former NFL linebacker Brian Bosworth admitted that he took caffeine pills before football games.

cross-country skiers perform at their peak for longer periods before they reach the point of exhaustion. Caffeine also helps athletes who must rely on quick reflexes, such as those who participate in such sports as baseball, basketball, tennis, fencing, football, soccer, boxing, and automobile racing. Studies conducted in 1975 and 1987 determined that caffeine enables athletes to react quicker.

Another clinical test of the effect of caffeine on athletes occurred during the late 1970s at the Human Performance Laboratory at Ball State University in Indiana. Those tests determined that as little as two hundred milligrams of caffeine could enhance an athlete's strength and endurance.

Caffeine Helps Provide Energy

There are a number of other ways caffeine provides an energy boost to athletes. For starters, caffeine enhances the circulation of "free fatty acids"—the chemicals metabolized from food that provide energy for the body. In other words, caffeine helps burn fatty acids quicker. When most people burn fatty acids beyond what they need for normal physical activity, they tend to lose weight. But when athletes take caffeine and burn fatty acids, they are generally in such good physical condition that there is no impact on their body weight. Instead, caffeine has other effects on athletes. By artificially speeding up the circulation of fatty acids in their bodies, athletes gain a new and powerful source of energy.

Caffeine also helps slow the body's depletion of the sugar glycogen, which is metabolized from such carbohydrate-rich foods as bread, pasta, and cereals. Glycogen is also an important source of energy for exercise; once glycogen is depleted from the body, exhaustion occurs and physical activity must stop. Because caffeine slows down the burn rate of glycogen, when athletes take caffeine their endurance improves.

Finally, caffeine is believed to have a psychological impact on athletes—it makes them feel stronger and more energetic. Most athletes would agree with the idea that in order to win, they must train their minds to believe they can win. If caffeine gives them mental as well as physical help, some will use it.

Breaking the Rules

Because of the performance-enhancing properties of caffeine, some athletes have come to rely on the drug as an integral part of their training. Brian Bosworth, a hard-hitting University of Oklahoma linebacker who later played professional football, said that prior to a game he typically consumed the equivalent of forty cups of coffee. Swimmer Sylvia Gerasch of Germany, who participated in many international competitions (including the 2000 Olympics), used caffeine before competitions. American Olympic cyclist Steve Hegg is reported to have consumed caffeine pills before his races. The Australian pentathalete Alex Watson used caffeine as well. Another Australian, rugby star George Gregan, said he used caffeine to help improve his performance during a game.

Those are famous names in athletic circles. However, several of them have gotten in trouble because of their caffeine use. Over the years, athletic organizations have prohibited caffeine from being used as a performance-enhancing drug. After Gerasch tested positive for caffeine in 1993, she was banned from international swimming competition for two years. Hegg won gold and silver medals at the 1984 Olympic Games in Los Angeles, but lost his place on the 1988 American cycling team when he tested positive for caffeine. Watson was also expelled from the 1988 Olympics for caffeine use.

Still, despite the occasional ban administered to caffeine-using athletes, caffeine does not face the widespread prohibition typical of other performance-enhancing substances, such as anabolic steroids. Currently, the National Collegiate Athletic Association (NCAA) is the lone major sports organization that regards caffeine as a "restricted substance." The NCAA will withdraw the eligibility of athletes who dope their bodies with caffeine prior to a competition.

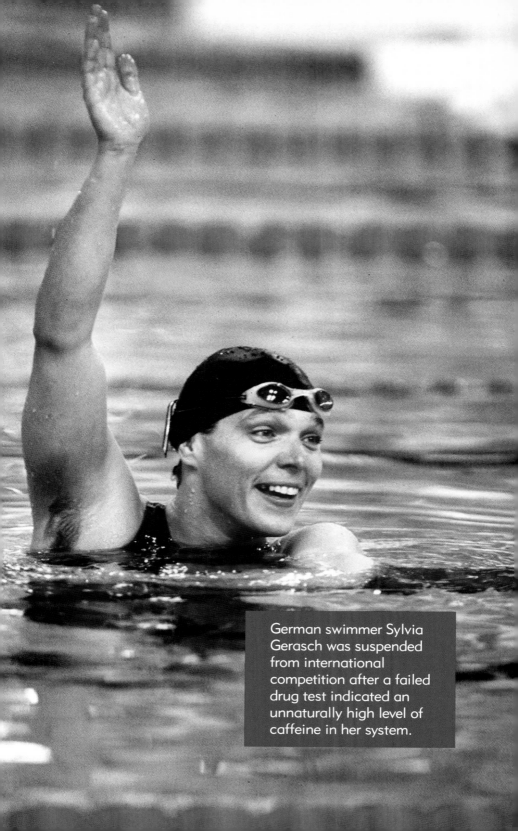

German swimmer Sylvia Gerasch was suspended from international competition after a failed drug test indicated an unnaturally high level of caffeine in her system.

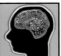
A 1998 study on caffeine and athletic performance determined that caffeine pills provide a better boost than coffee or caffeinated drinks. As part of the study, long-distance runners consumed pills containing three hundred milligrams of caffeine—about the equivalent of two cups of coffee—and were then sent out to run as fast and as far as they could until they reached the point of exhaustion. Next, the runners were given the same task after simply drinking coffee containing the same levels of caffeine. The study found that the runners covered longer distances at a faster pace after consuming the caffeine pills.

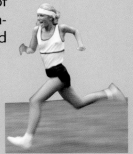

Studies show that caffeine pills are more effective than coffee at enhancing workouts.

Why did the runners do better on pure caffeine than on an equal dose of caffeinated coffee? Evidently, there are other ingredients in coffee that impede athletic performance. In a separate study, Vanderbilt University professor Peter R. Martin found that coffee contains chlorogenic acids that add to the aroma of the bean but also deaden the stimulating effects of caffeine. Researchers Bennett Alan Weinberg and Bonnie K. Bealer wrote, "If Martin is right, they may be the culprits that work to limit the power of caffeine when it is delivered by coffee. Tea also contains chlorogenic acids, so it may interfere with caffeine as well."

Bennett Alan Weinberg and Bonnie K. Bealer, *The Caffeine Advantage*. New York: Free Press, 2002, p. 134.

Although in the past the International Olympic Committee (IOC) has banned athletes for caffeine use, the organization no longer regards caffeine as a prohibited substance. The IOC's decision to permit or ban a particular substance is based on judgments made by the World Anti-Doping Agency; this agency, which is based in Montreal, was formed in 1999. Representatives from eighty-one nations as well as sixty-two international sports organizations have agreed to abide by the World Anti-Doping Agency's recommendations. Each year, the World Anti-Doping Agency reviews the medical impacts and performance-enhancing qualities of substances and decides which drugs should not be used by athletes who participate in international competitions, such as the Olympics.

At one time, caffeine was on the agency's list of banned substances, but the organization removed it from the list in 2004. The primary reason for caffeine's removal was that, in the view of the organization, tests of athletes for evidence of caffeine abuse were unreliable. But there are other questions surrounding prohibitions and testing as well. Can a substance that is legal be prohibited from consumption? Also, how much of a substance should be considered too much?

"Bordering on Cheating"

Most drug tests are conducted through an analysis of urine. If an athlete has consumed an anabolic steroid, a tiny amount will show up in the sample—a positive test. Anabolic steroids are generally available only through prescription, so most athletes must acquire them illegally. A positive test that violates an anti-steroid ban imposed by a sporting organization means the athlete faces a ban or other punishment.

When caffeine shows up in a urine sample, however, the user's guilt is not as easy to determine. Unlike anabolic steroids, caffeine is a legal substance that is available in many commonly consumed beverages. The tested athlete may have consumed only a few cups of coffee before taking the test.

Athletic organizations must also determine how much caffeine gives an athlete an artificial advantage. At one time, the IOC banned athletes whose urine contained more than fourteen micrograms of caffeine per milliliter (a microgram is one-millionth of a gram; a milliliter is equal to one thousandth of a liter), believing this would provide them an unfair athletic advantage. The NCAA continues to ban athletes with urine tests containing more than fifteen micrograms of caffeine per milliliter. Scientific tests have shown those levels are virtually impossible to reach under natural conditions. For example, even test subjects who consumed ten cups of coffee shortly before providing the urine sample did not achieve this level of caffeine saturation in their urine.

Although the World Anti-Doping Agency has removed caffeine from its list of banned substances, in 2005 the agency said it was considering putting caffeine back on its banned list. At the time, David Howman, the director-general of the World Anti-Doping Agency, told ABC Premium News of Australia that caffeine use by athletes is "bordering on cheating. If it's not on the list it's not cheating, but it's bordering. . . . Each sport's got to be in a position, whether it determines that's acceptable for it or not. I think society's got to make that same sort of decision."[36]

A Dangerous Combination

Aside from the question of whether caffeine doping should be considered cheating, a more serious problem has emerged involving caffeine use by athletes. In recent years, some American companies have begun producing over-the-counter supplements that contain both caffeine and the herb ephedra. (Typically, in dietary supplements the caffeine is supplied by another herb, guarana.) Ephedra affects the body in ways similar to caffeine, and has also been shown to enhance athletic performance. As a result, some athletes began using the caffeine-ephedra combination, believing it would improve their workouts.

That is what Sean Riggins believed. A high school wrestler and football player in Lincoln, Illinois, Sean prepared for each competition by swallowing a dietary supplement known as Yellow Jacket that includes both ephedra and caffeine. He often washed down the pill with a tall glass of Mountain Dew or Red Bull. The caffeine and ephedra seemed to make him incredibly strong: at the age of sixteen, weighing just 170 pounds, Sean could dead-lift 425 pounds.

Shortly before a football game in the fall of 2002, Sean told his coach he did not feel well. The next morning, he saw a doctor who, after being assured by the teenager that he had not taken any drugs, diagnosed Sean's condition as the flu. That afternoon, Sean Riggins suffered a heart attack and died. Because it is highly unusual for a very healthy and athletic teenager to die from a heart attack, Lincoln coroner Chuck Fricke ordered an autopsy. "Basically his heart was pumping

Diet pills that contain both caffeine and ephedra have been linked to the deaths of several athletes. (Ephedrine, listed on the label below, is the active ingredient in the herb ephedra.)

so fast, it gave out on him,"[37] Fricke told a reporter for *Sports Illustrated*.

Although the autopsy did not test for caffeine and ephedra, when Sean's father learned that his son had been taking the dietary supplement, he knew no other tests would be necessary. "After we heard he had taken ephedra, it all made sense," Kevin Riggins told *Sports Illustrated*. "As much sense as you can make of having an active, athletic 16-year-old one day and then having him drop dead the next."[38]

Other athletes have also died after using products containing ephedra and caffeine. In 2001, Minnesota Vikings lineman Korey Stringer died of heatstroke during training camp. In 2003, Baltimore Orioles pitcher Steve Bechler died from heatstroke during spring training. Both athletes had been using ephedra-based dietary supplements. Following their

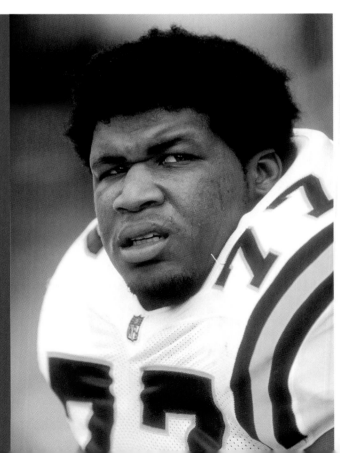

A product containing caffeine and ephedra may have contributed to the death of Korey Stringer, an offensive tackle for the Minnesota Vikings.

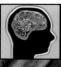 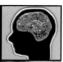

Caffeine and Dehydration

Athletes who consume caffeine before a workout should be mindful that the drug can cause dehydration. This can be particularly hazardous, because high-intensity workouts cause people to lose body fluids rapidly through perspiration. That is why athletes who consume caffeine should also be sure to drink plenty of water during their workouts.

Dehydration, said authors Bennett Alan Weinberg and Bonnie K. Bealer in their book *The World of Caffeine: The Science and Culture of the World's Most Popular Drug*, is "one of the primary problems for athletes, especially endurance athletes, because the fatigue experienced as a result of dehydration is indistinguishable from the normal fatigue of hard training."

However, one caffeine-related issue that long-distance runners, cross-country skiers, cyclists, and other athletes who use the drug should not have to worry about is frequent urination. Although caffeine is a diuretic and therefore enhances urination, an article published in the March 1, 2000, issue of the *Journal of Sports Medicine and Physical Fitness* reported that exercise helps stall the kidneys' release of fluid.

The same article warned, however, that athletes who consume caffeine could experience cramping. Most athletic trainers, however, know how to cure cramping—by having athletes drink plenty of water, something they need to do anyway.

Bennett Alan Weinberg and Bonnie K. Bealer, *The World of Caffeine: The Science and Culture of the World's Most Popular Drug*. New York: Routledge, 2002, p. 222.

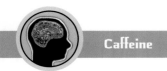

deaths, the U.S. Food and Drug Administration issued a ban on ephedra-based dietary supplements. However, the ban was lifted on April 15, 2005, by a federal judge in Utah, who ruled that the FDA had failed to present enough evidence showing ephedra could be dangerous.

Today, many doctors and nutritionists suggest that athletes should avoid ingesting supplements that contain ephedra and guarana. However, some physical fitness experts insist that athletes can use caffeine safely and effectively. For example, in a February 1, 2003, article in the magazine *Joe Weider's Shape*, science editor Jim Stoppani recommended reducing caffeine intake during times of the day other than workout times. This allows the athlete to save his or her caffeine jolt for the workout, when it will provide the greatest benefit. "Studies show that people who aren't regular caffeine consumers get much better results than regular users and need significantly smaller amounts of it," he said.[39] Also, Stoppani suggested, for the best results an athlete should consume just two hundred to three hundred milligrams of caffeine within two hours of the workout. That amounts to no more than a couple of cups of coffee.

Energy Drinks

Athletes who avoid dietary supplements may prefer to consume their caffeine in the form of energy drinks, such as Red Bull, Killer Buzz, Full Throttle, and Rip It. The names clearly indicate the purpose of these drinks: an energy boost for consumers. Some of these drinks include guarana, a caffeine-containing plant; others contain both guarana and caffeine, meaning they provide a double dose of the drug.

Nutritionists agree that energy drinks are poor substitutes for the fuel that provides the body with the best form of energy—a balanced and healthy diet. In an interview with a *Seattle Times* reporter, University of Maryland nutrition professor Mark Kanter said, "These drinks are marketing ploys. I'm not aware of any scientific data that they do what they say they're going to do. They don't give you more energy. . . . A nutritionist defines energy as calories. If you refer to energy as something that gives you pep and zip and stamina, that's just a myth."[40]

Yet some companies aggressively market their products to young people. One of these is a drink called KickStart Spark, which contains sixty milligrams of caffeine and is targeted for young athletes—even children as young as four years. A website advertising this product is headlined "KickStart Kids" and features photographs of young athletes running races on a track, competing in martial arts competitions, and skateboarding. According to the website, "Whether it's at the game, on the playground or in the classroom, your child needs KickStart Spark for better energy and focus."[41]

Despite the concerns of nutritionists, AdvoCare International, the company that manufactures KickStart Spark, has defended its product. Company executive Sidney Stohs told the *New York Times* in 2005, "It's not just a caffeine delivery system; it has many more nutritional properties."[42] According to the company's website, the beverage "contains 20 vitamins, minerals, and nutrients that keep your child healthy."[43]

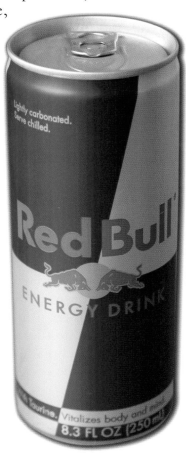

Red Bull is among the most popular of the highly caffeinated energy drinks on the market today.

Nevertheless, pediatricians told the *New York Times* that more research must be performed on caffeine and its effects on children and adolescents before they would feel comfortable letting young people consume caffeine in such large quantities. Pediatrician Mary L. Gavin warned, "Their little bodies handle it differently, and they don't need it. It's a stimulant. The likelihood that a child is going to have side effects is much higher at that age."[44]

Others believe giving caffeine to young athletes sends a bad message. They suggest that if a parent or coach hands a child an energy drink and recommends that the child consume it before a game, it is likely that when the athlete grows older he or she may seek out more dangerous substances, such as anabolic steroids. Frank Uryasz, president of the National Center for Drug Free Sport, told the *New York Times* that young athletes should avoid caffeine. "I am concerned that they are gateway substances," he said. "I think it develops a mind-set especially among young athletes that they have to take something—a powder, a pill, a liquid—to improve their performance, when actually study after study shows that almost all of these products add no value to a young person's athletic performance."[45]

No One Really Needs Caffeine

Many athletes prefer to play the game without performance-enhancing drugs, and find they can compete on a high level without them. In fact, no one really needs caffeine. Today, it is not difficult to find caffeine-free beverages and products at the supermarket. But people who wish to lead caffeine-free lives need to do more than just consume the right products. They need to break out of a social atmosphere that encourages them to be constantly stimulated by caffeine.

Chapter 5

LIVING A CAFFEINE-FREE LIFE

Caffeine has become such a way of life among some people that it is hard for them to imagine what life might be like without the drug. Still, there are alternatives to caffeine. Nearly every beverage that contains caffeine can be substituted with a decaffeinated or even naturally caffeine-free selection. By doing a little homework, reading the labels, and selecting products carefully, it is possible for anyone to live a caffeine-free life.

Hard to Avoid

Clearly, caffeine use is on the rise in the United States, Europe, and many other places around the world. People of all ages enjoy coffee, tea, soft drinks, and other caffeinated products, and annual sales of these products total tens of billions of dollars. "Today, more than any time before, caffeine is the dominant, nearly universal drug of the human race," Weinberg and Bealer wrote in *The World of Caffeine*:

> It was in the steaming cups of coffee or tea that sat alongside the men who created the first newspapers. It

is in the steaming cups of coffee or tea or, nearly as often, in the cold colas or other carbonated soft drinks that sit by those who design and use the Internet software and websites that are taking us into the third millennium.

Other drugs have had their days, for the use of many intoxicants is cyclic, rising and falling over the decades and centuries. Certainly caffeine use has not remained constant, nor can it be absolutely asserted that its use has demonstrated an unbroken increase in every nation in every decade. Yet, during the five centuries since word of the caffeinated beverages reached Europe, the coffee bean alone has come to account for a greater share of international trade than any other agricultural commodity, and these beverages have reached every quarter of every country on the earth.[46]

Caffeinated beverages can be found everywhere. For example, small coffee shops can be found throughout the town of Chapel Hill, home to the sprawling campus of the Univer-

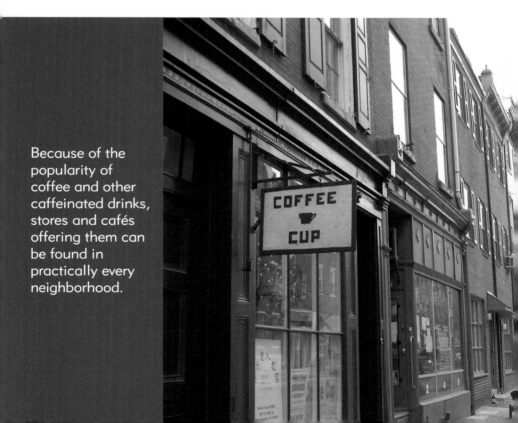

Because of the popularity of coffee and other caffeinated drinks, stores and cafés offering them can be found in practically every neighborhood.

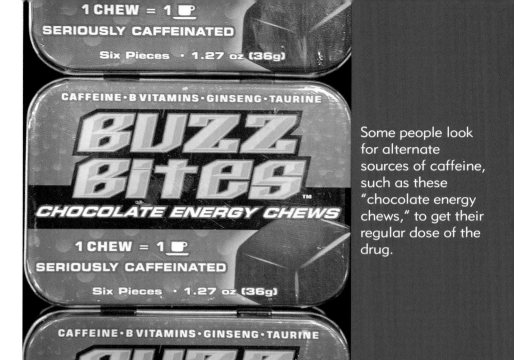

Some people look for alternate sources of caffeine, such as these "chocolate energy chews," to get their regular dose of the drug.

sity of North Carolina (UNC). "College towns and coffee shops go hand in hand," Grant Meadows, manager of one such establishment, told the *Daily Tar Heel* in 2005. "Our society is becoming more and more inundated with coffee."[47] At Meadows' coffee shop, the percolators boil one-hundred pounds of coffee grounds a week, brewing thousands of cups which are primarily consumed by UNC students.

But students do not even have to step off campus to find coffee. UNC students who study at the school's Health Sciences Library can take a coffee break at the Friends Café, located right in the library. Matt Dallas, a shift supervisor at the café, told *Daily Tar Heel* reporter Linda Shen that both students and faculty members work long hours in the library, and they clearly seem to need a caffeine jolt from time to time to help them stay awake and alert. "The people who come in aren't really people," he said. "They're machines trained to drink all our coffee."[48] The Friends Café brews as much as 125 pots of regular coffee a week as well as thirty-five pots of flavored gourmet coffee.

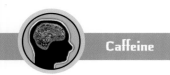

Across the Atlantic Ocean, *National Geographic* writer T.R. Reid discovered the latest caffeine trend circulating among the dancers at London's all-night dance clubs. Previously, after dancing for hours to the frenzied pace of rave music, dancers found themselves tiring around four o'clock in the morning. But then they discovered Red Bull and the other energy drinks. Simon Patrick, manager of the Egg nightclub in London, told Reid, "Actually, we usually see a revival about half-past four or so in the morning. That's when we get the real rush at the bar for Red Bull. And the kids say, 'I've had eight Red Bulls—I'm flying!' They'll dance right round the clock. At seven in the morning we have trouble getting them out the door." Added Neil Stanley, director of sleep research at the Human Psychopharmacology Research Unit at Great Britain's University of Surrey, "The kids in the clubs, they think they've happened upon this great new invention. But we've known for centuries that caffeinated drinks work. They get you out of an energy slump and make you more alert. Really all they've found is a new kind of caffeine delivery system."[49]

Caffeine-Free Products Available

But in the midst of this modern caffeine craze, some people are deciding that they want to cut back or eliminate their consumption of this drug. To find caffeine-free products, consumers need only take the time to do a little detective work. There are many caffeine-free soft drinks on the market that taste similar to the caffeinated versions. For example, both Pepsi-Cola and Coca-Cola sell caffeine-free versions of their popular products, and other companies manufacture caffeine-free soft drinks as well. In 2003, *Consumer Reports* magazine conducted a blind taste test using children to assess caffeinated and caffeine-free soft drinks. The magazine reported, "We've found that many kids did not prefer regular to caffeine-free versions of the same soda, and some kids actually liked the caffeine-free versions better."[50]

In addition, many carbonated soft drinks have never contained caffeine. The popular soft drink 7-Up has been around since 1929. It contains no caffeine. Similar drinks like Fresca and Sprite are also caffeine free, and most root beers and ginger ales do not contain the drug.

There are also decaffeinated beverages, in which practically all of the caffeine has been removed from a product that ordinarily contains the drug. Decaffeinated coffee has been on the market since 1906, when German inventor Ludwig Roselius perfected the decaffeination process. Essentially, Roselius soaked coffee beans in water, then exposed them to a chemical solvent to leach out most of the caffeine. In the 1970s, German researchers developed an improved method of decaffeinating coffee by using carbon dioxide to remove the caffeine from the beans. Most American coffee companies have adopted this method or similar processes so that chemicals are no longer used.

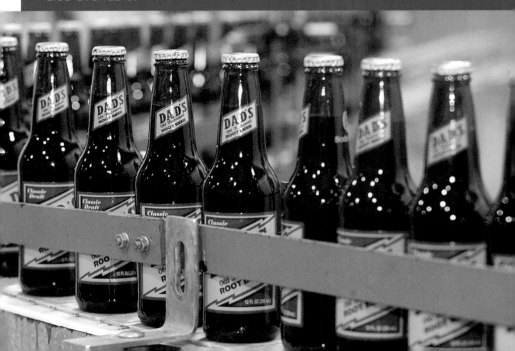

Some sodas, such as root beer, are naturally free from caffeine. In addition, caffeine-free versions of many popular drinks are also available.

But no matter what method is used to create decaffeinated coffee, the end result is not completely caffeine free—usually, three to five milligrams of caffeine remain in a cup of decaf coffee. Still, that is considerably less than the caffeine found in a cup of regular coffee.

Tea generally has less caffeine than coffee. It can be relatively easy for the tea drinker to control the amount of caffeine he or she ingests simply by shortening the amount of time a tea bag soaks in the hot water. The longer the bag soaks, the more caffeine is transferred from the leaves to the drink. Caffeine-free and decaffeinated teas are also available on the market. The caffeine in tea is removed using a carbon dioxide process similar to that used to decaffeinate coffee. Herbal teas are naturally caffeine-free, because they are not made from the leaves of the tea plant (*Camellia sinensis*).

While there are many caffeine-free and decaffeinated beverages, chocolate has yet to be made in a caffeine-free or decaffeinated form. Still, some chocolate products contain more caffeine than others. A 1.4-ounce serving of dark chocolate,

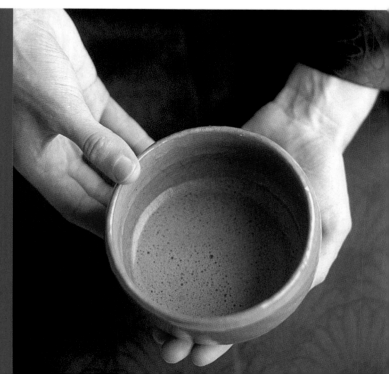

Green tea and other herbal tees are available for those who want to avoid ingesting caffeine.

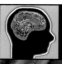 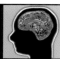

There are beverages that are alternatives to coffee that are made from cereal grains and other natural ingredients and do not contain caffeine. One of the first such beverages, Postum, was developed in 1895 by cereal maker Charles William Post, who believed that caffeine was unhealthy.

Postum's ingredients include wheat, bran, and molasses, but Post insisted that his concoction tasted just like coffee if made correctly. "When well brewed," Post claimed, "Postum has the deep seal brown of coffee and a flavor very like the milder brands of Java."

Today, Postum is manufactured by Kraft Foods and can be found in most major supermarkets.

Quoted in Mark Pendergrast, *Uncommon Grounds.* New York: Basic Books, 1999, p. 99.

for example, contains twenty-eight milligrams of caffeine, which puts it in the same league with some soft drinks and teas. A similar serving of milk chocolate, on the other hand, contains much less caffeine—between three and ten milligrams. One way to avoid caffeine while still enjoying the taste of chocolate is to eat a piece of chocolate-coated candy rather than a bar of pure chocolate.

Drinking decaffeinated coffee or tea or caffeine-free soft drinks are easy ways a person can cut down on his or her caffeine intake. However, completely avoiding caffeine can be a challenge. Hundreds of products available on supermarket shelves contain caffeine, yet their labels may not reveal that fact. Because the U.S. Food and Drug Administration considers caffeine a safe drug, it has ruled that a product's caffeine content only has to be listed on the label if the caffeine

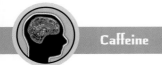

has been artificially added. Even then, the manufacturer is not required to report the amount of caffeine that has been added, just note that the product is caffeine-enhanced.

Making Caffeine Content Public

Consumer organizations have lobbied the FDA, hoping to convince the agency that providing information on caffeine content to shoppers would help people understand the health consequences of consuming the drug. In 1997, the Washington-based Center for Science in the Public Interest presented a seventy-page petition to Congress calling for lawmakers to require caffeine labeling on products. Among the signers of the petition were thirty-four scientists and representatives from ten health care and consumer groups. In a news release, Michael Jacobson, executive director of the organization, said, "Caffeine is the only drug that is widely added to the food supply, and consumers have a right to know how much caffeine various foods contain. Knowing the caffeine content is important to many people—especially women who are or might become pregnant—who might want to limit or avoid caffeine."[51]

Congress has held hearings on this issue. In 2004, Lester Crawford, the acting commissioner of the FDA, testified before the House Appropriations Committee's Subcommittee on Agriculture. He insisted that many scientific studies have been conducted on caffeine but that there is hardly a consensus in the scientific community on whether caffeine is truly harmful to human health. Without significant scientific evidence that definitely shows the health impact of caffeine on the body, Crawford said, the FDA would find itself unable to fight a court challenge against caffeine labeling that would likely be brought by a coffee or soft drink company. Crawford testified,

> One paper comes out, and it's the worst thing on the earth. Another paper comes out that shows it has only transient effects on the heart, which is the major target

CAFFEINE CONTENT OF SELECTED PRODUCTS

Product	Serving Size	Caffeine (mg)
OTC DRUGS		
NoDoz, max. strength, Vivarin	1 tablet	200
Excedrin	2 tablets	130
COFFEES		
Coffee, brewed	8 ounces	135
Coffee, instant	8 ounces	95
Maxwell House Cappuchino, Mocha	8 ounces	60-65
Maxwell House Cappuchino, decaffeinated	8 ounces	3-6
Coffee, decaffeinated	8 ounces	5
TEAS		
Tea, leaf or bag	8 ounces	50
Lipton Iced Tea, assorted varieties	16-ounce bottle	18-40
Tea, green	8 ounces	30
Tea, instant	8 ounces	15
Celestial Seasonings Herbal Tea, all varieties	8 ounces	0
SOFT DRINKS		
Mountain Dew	12 ounces	55.5
Diet Coke	12 ounces	46.5
Coca-Cola Classic	12 ounces	34.5
Dr. Pepper, regular or diet	12 ounces	42
Pepsi-Cola	12 ounces	37.5
7-UP or Diet 7-UP	12 ounces	0
Caffeine-free Coca-Cola or Diet Coke	12 ounces	0
Caffeine-free Pepsi or Diet Pepsi	12 ounces	0
CAFFEINATED WATER		
Java Water	16.9 ounces	125
Water Joe	16.9 ounces	90
CHOCOLATES/CANDIES		
Hershey's Special Dark Chocolate Bar	1 bar (1.5 ounces)	31
Hershey Bar (milk chocolate)	1 bar (1.5 ounces)	10
Cocoa or Hot Chocolate	8 ounces	5

Sources: National Coffee Association, National Soft Drink Association, Tea Council of the USA, and information provided by food, beverage, and pharmaceutical companies and J.J. Barone, H.R. Roberts (1996) "Caffeine Consumption." *Food Chemistry and Toxicology,* vol. 34, pp. 119–129.

organ. And so, in terms of whether we could enforce limiting caffeine based on the science and the current state of medical scientific understanding of it, is what's at odds. Right now, it looks like caffeine is safer than was previously understood.[52]

Because it appears unlikely that the FDA will require food packagers to include caffeine content on their labels any time

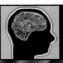 **Tips on Cutting Down**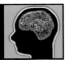

In his book *Caffeine Blues*, nutritionist Stephen Cherniske offered tips for caffeine users looking for ways to cut down their consumption of the drug. For example, he suggested one way to cut down is to combine decaffeinated and regular coffee before brewing. Cherniske recommended starting with a fifty-fifty mix, then gradually increasing the decaf content until the coffee drinker is consuming decaf only. Other suggestions include brewing a weaker pot of coffee (using more water and less coffee) or adding more milk or cream to the cup.

One simple way to reduce the amount of caffeine consumed is to drink smaller amounts of the beverage. Cherniske recalled treating a client who complained that she was having trouble getting a good night's sleep. The difficulty started soon after her thirtieth birthday. At first, Cherniske said, the client chalked up her sleep troubles to just getting older, then realized that the real problem was a very large coffee mug she had been given as a present. By using the new mug, she was inadvertently ingesting more caffeine than normal.

soon, consumers are on their own if they wish to find out the caffeine levels that exist in the coffee, soft drinks, and other products they eat or drink. That information is not hard to find—anyone with access to the Internet can learn the caffeine content of hundreds of products very quickly.

Comparing Products

There are many websites that list the caffeine content of food and beverage products. The websites providing this information are maintained by manufacturers, trade associations, health organizations, and consumer watchdog groups. With a little research, a consumer can learn, for instance, that a serving of Ben & Jerry's No Fat Coffee Fudge Frozen Yogurt contains 86 milligrams of caffeine while a serving of Häagen-Dazs fat-free Coffee Frozen Yogurt contains 40 milligrams of caffeine. Here are two very similar products, and yet one contains less than half the caffeine of the other.

People who want to avoid caffeine or cut down on their use of the drug must become educated consumers. One of the best places to begin looking for caffeine content is the website of the American Beverage Association at www.ameribev.org. The organization serves as a trade association for major soft drink manufacturers and has made information available on the caffeine content of its members' beverages. Also, several soft drink makers have listed the caffeine content of their products on their own websites, including Pepsi-Cola at www.pepsi.com and Coca-Cola at www.cocacola.com. Hershey's, the manufacturer of several chocolate products, lists the caffeine content of its candies and desserts at www.hersheys.com. Consumer groups, such as the Center for Science in the Public Interest at www.cspint.org, and health organizations, including the Mayo Clinic in Rochester, Minnesota, at www.mayoclinic.org, have compiled their own lists of caffeinated products.

Consumer experts agree that parents who do the food shopping for their households should also be educated about products and their caffeine content. Said Consumers Union president Jim Guest, "Parents often don't know that there is caffeine in many of the products they buy, and many products don't disclose the presence of caffeine unless they've added it in and, even then, they don't disclose how much is in there."[53]

Making Intelligent Decisions

Although the Food and Drug Administration has chosen not to act on caffeine labeling, other organizations have taken steps to help young people learn about unhealthy diets. For several years, many school boards authorized the installation of vending machines in school cafeterias as a way to raise revenue. In recent years, though, some school administrators are rethinking their policies and have ordered the machines removed. Certainly, these actions were taken primarily in response to the obesity epidemic among young people because most products sold in vending machines have high fat and sugar contents. Nevertheless, soft drinks, coffee, and chocolate candies are typically sold in vending machines as well, so by taking all the machines out of schools, administrators have also removed sources of caffeine. Some schools have removed caffeine from the lunchroom as well, by banning the sale of soft drinks in school cafeterias.

Janette Faul, a spokesperson for Peak Performance, a Wisconsin-based organization that works with schools on nutrition issues, told *Education Week* magazine, "One of the reasons students drink so much soda is that it's a meal supplement. Many students have to get up early to go to school, [and] they're not hungry when they get up to get to the bus, so when they get to school they go to vending machines."[54]

Nutritionists, consumerism experts, physicians, and others believe that it is important for young people to become educated consumers, so they can learn how to use caffeine products in safe and moderate amounts. Many advocate limiting youngsters' caffeine consumption, and believe schools have

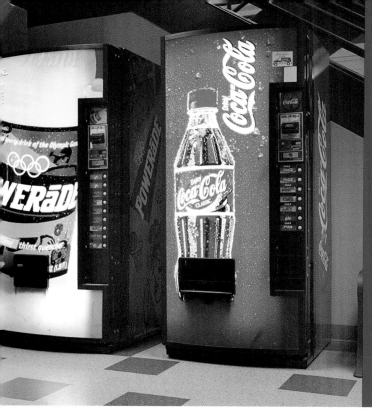

In recent years, some school districts have begun removing vending machines that offer caffeinated soft drinks. Other districts have stopped selling such drinks in their cafeterias.

not been active enough in this process. Marcia Rubin, director of research for the American School Health Association, told *Education Week*, "I think schools should do a better job of explaining what caffeine can do to your body and limiting kids' access to it."[55]

In proper quantities, caffeine may provide many benefits to human health, enhance athletic performance, make the mind sharper, and provide an energy boost. But even caffeine's most dedicated proponents will admit that it is an addictive drug that affects its users both physically and mentally. Understanding the levels of caffeine in foods and beverages, and the substance's effects on the body and brain, will help people make intelligent decisions about whether they want to use this drug.

NOTES

Introduction: The World's Most Popular Drug

1. National Public Radio, "Interview: Bennett Alan Weinberg discusses the discovery of caffeine, the significant amounts consumed daily, and the book he co-authored, *The World of Caffeine*," *Weekend Edition Saturday*, September 8, 2001.

Chapter 1: Caffeine Through the Ages

2. Quoted in Jill Norman, *Coffee*. New York: Bantam Books, 1992, p. 8.
3. Quoted in Bennett Alan Weinberg and Bonnie K. Bealer, *The World of Caffeine: The Science and Culture of the World's Most Popular Drug*. New York: Routledge, 2002, p. 166.
4. Quoted in Weinberg and Bealer, *The World of Caffeine*, p. 121.
5. T.R. Reid, "What's the Buzz?" *National Geographic*, January 1, 2005, p. 2.
6. Quoted in Frederick Allen, *Secret Formula: How Brilliant Marketing and Relentless Salesmanship Made Coca-Cola the Best-Known Product in the World*. New York: HarperBusiness, 1994, p. 61.
7. National Public Radio, "The Coffee Break," *Morning Edition*, December 2, 2002. www.npr.org/programs/morning/features/patc/coffeebreak.
8. Edward M. Brecher, *Licit and Illicit Drugs*. Mount Vernon, N.Y.: Consumers Union, 1972, p. 201.
9. National Public Radio, interview with Bennett Alan Weinberg, *Weekend Edition Saturday*, September 8, 2001.

Chapter 2: How Caffeine Impacts Human Health

10. Quoted in Edward M. Brecher, *Licit and Illicit Drugs*. Mount Vernon, N.Y.: Consumers Union, 1972, p. 199.

11. Stephen Chernieske, *Caffeine Blues: Wake Up to the Hidden Dangers of America's No. 1 Drug*. New York: Warner Books, 1998, p. 81.

12. Charles P. Pollack and David Bright, "Caffeine Consumption and Weekly Sleep Patterns in U.S. Seventh-, Eighth-, and Ninth-Graders," *Pediatrics*, January 1, 2003, p. 42.

13. Chernieske, *Caffeine Blues*, p. 222.

14. Weinberg and Bealer, *The World of Caffeine*, p. 314.

15. Jeremy Pawloski, "Report Blames Caffeine OD in Mom's Death," *Albuquerque Journal*, November 30, 2004, p. A3.

16. National Public Radio, "Caffeine Consumption Linked to Miscarriage," *Morning Edition*, December 22, 1993.

17. Stephen Braun, *Buzz: The Science and Lore of Alcohol and Caffeine*. New York: Penguin, 1996, p. 112.

Chapter 3: Addicted to Caffeine

18. Judy Monroe, "Caffeine's Hook," *Current Health 2*, January 1, 1998, p. 16.

19. Anne Neville, "Fill 'er Up: Coffee Is the Jolt that Fuels the Day for Local Caffeine Junkies Hot on the Trail of a Fix," *Buffalo News*, August 28, 2005. p. B-1.

20. Neville, "Fill 'er Up," p. B-1.

21. Mark Pendergrast, *Uncommon Grounds*. New York: Basic Books, 1999, p. 416.

22. Monroe, "Caffeine's Hook," p. 16.

23. Weinberg and Bealer, *The World of Caffeine*, p. 305.

24. Pendergrast, *Uncommon Grounds*, p. 416.

25. Monroe, "Caffeine's Hook," p. 16.

26. Bennett Alan Weinberg and Bonnie K. Bealer, *The Caffeine Advantage*. New York: Free Press, 2002, p. 29.

27. Dana Sullivan, "Wake Me Up: A Cup of Coffee to Kick Start Your Day Won't Harm Your Health," *Real Simple*, December 1, 2004, p. 163.

28. Weinberg and Bealer, *The Caffeine Advantage*, p. 30.

29. Weinberg and Bealer, *The World of Caffeine*, p. 306.

30. CBS News Early Show, "Kicking the Caffeine Habit," February 25, 2005. www.cbsnews.com/stories/2005/02/24/earlyshow/living/ConsumerWatch/main676309.shtml.
31. CBS News Early Show, "Kicking the Caffeine Habit."
32. CBS News Early Show, "Kicking the Caffeine Habit."
33. Janet Brigham, *Dying to Quit: Why We Smoke and How We Stop*. Washington: Joseph Henry Press, 1998, pp. 120–21.
34. Weinberg and Bealer, *The World of Caffeine*, p. 276.

Chapter 4: Caffeine and Sports

35. Rick Telander, "The Big Enchilada: Tony Mandarich, a Top NFL Prospect, Is a Chowhound Who Chews Up Opponents," *Sports Illustrated*, April 24, 1989. http://sportsillustrated.cnn.com/2004/pr/subs/siexclusive/07/08/flashback.mandarich/index.html
36. Rob Cross, "Caffeine Use 'Bordering on Cheating': WADA," ABC Premium News, May 18, 2005. http://www.abc.net.au/sport/content/200505/s1371529.htm
37. L. John Wertheim, "Jolt of Reality: Following the Lead of Elite Athletes, Teenagers Are Increasingly Juicing Their Workouts with Pills and Powders—Sometimes with Tragic Results," *Sports Illustrated*, April 7, 2003, p. 68.
38. Wertheim, "Jolt of Reality," p. 68.
39. Jim Stoppani, "Caffeine + Exercise = Fat Loss," *Joe Weider's Shape*, February 1, 2003, p. 36.
40. Ari Bloomekatz, "Medical Experts Warn of Unhealthy Buzz-Touting Energy Drinks," *Seattle Times*, August 15, 2005. http://seattletimes.nwsource.com/html/health/2002430338_healthenergy10.html
41. AdvoCare International, "KickStart Kids." www.advocare.com/store/getProductDetail.do?itemCode=K2083&id=H.
42. Duff Wilson, "A Sports Drink for Children Is Jangling Some Nerves," *New York Times*, September 25, 2005, p. H-1.

43. AdvoCare International, "KickStart Spark." www.advo care.com/store/getProductDetail.do?itemCode=K2083&i d=H.

44. Wilson, "A Sports Drink for Children Is Jangling Some Nerves," p. H-1.

45. Wilson, "A Sports Drink for Children Is Jangling Some Nerves," p. H-1.

Chapter 5: Living a Caffeine-Free Life

46. Weinberg and Bealer, *The World of Caffeine*, pp. 319–20.

47. Linda Shen, "Campus Buzzing for Caffeine," *The Daily Tar Heel*, September 21, 2005. www.dailytarheel.com/vnews /display.v/ART/2005/09/21/4330d92879ed7.

48. Shen, "Campus Buzzing for Caffeine."

49. Reid, "What's the Buzz?", p. 2.

50. *Consumer Reports*, "Caffeinated Kids," July 1, 2003. http://www.consumerreports.org/cro/babies-kids/caffein ated-kids-703/overview.htm

51. Center for Science in the Public Interest, "Label Caffeine Content on Foods, Scientists Tell FDA," July 31, 1997. www.cspint.org/new/caffeine.htm.

52. U.S. House Committee on Appropriations: Subcommittee on Agriculture, "Hearing on the FY05 Appropriations for Programs Under its Jurisdiction: Testimony of Lester M. Crawford, D.V.M., Ph.D., Acting Commissioner, Food and Drug Administration, Department of Health and Human Services" March 11, 2004.

53. Zachery Kouwe, "Here's a Jolt: Caffeine Exists Where It Often Isn't Expected," *Wall Street Journal*, June 10, 2003, p. D-8.

54. Marianne D. Hurst, "Caffeine's Impact on Students Cited in Push to Curb School Drink Sales," *Education Week*, March 12, 2003, p. 38.

55. Hurst, "Caffeine's Impact on Students Cited in Push to Curb School Drink Sales," p. 38.

ORGANIZATIONS TO CONTACT

Center for Science in the Public Interest
1875 Connecticut Ave. NW, Suite 300
Washington, DC 20009
(202) 332-9110
http://www.cspinet.org/new/caffeine.htm

This consumer group has called for federal legislation requiring food and beverage companies to include caffeine content on labels. The organization has posted on its website the caffeine content of many foods and beverages available in American stores.

Mayo Clinic
200 First St. SW
Rochester, MN 55905
(507) 284-2511
http://www.mayoclinic.com/health/caffeine/AN00549

The world-famous Mayo Clinic has posted a number of articles assessing the safety of caffeine use on its Web site, which also includes the caffeine content of some of the most commonly consumed foods and beverages in the United States.

National Coffee Association
15 Maiden Lane, Suite 1405
New York, NY 10038
(212) 766-4007
http://www.ncausa.org
http://coffeescience.org

The National Coffee Association is a trade group of American coffee companies.

U. S. Food and Drug Administration
5600 Fishers Lane
Rockville, MD 20857-0001
(888) 463-6332
http://www.fda.gov
The federal agency charged with regulating the safety of foods, beverages, and drugs in the American marketplace has issued a number of reports and advisories on caffeine, particularly when it is employed as an ingredient in dietary supplements that also include the herb ephedra.

World Anti-Doping Agency
Stock Exchange Tower
800 Place Victoria, Suite 1700
PO Box 120
Montreal, Quebec H4Z 1B7
Canada
(514) 904-9232
http://www.wada-ama.org/en

The organization issues an annual list of substances that are banned from use by athletes in international competitions. Through publications and conferences, the World Anti-Doping Agency also provides educational and outreach programs to help alert athletes about the dangers of performance-enhancing substances.

FOR MORE INFORMATION

Books

Frederick Allen, *Secret Formula: How Brilliant Marketing and Relentless Salesmanship Made Coca-Cola the Best-Known Product in the World*. New York: HarperBusiness, 1994. A complete history of one of America's most familiar soft drinks, the book includes an examination of the 1911 trial, which the U.S. government hoped would result in banning caffeine as an ingredient of soft drinks.

Stephen Braun, *Buzz: The Science and Lore of Alcohol and Caffeine*. New York: Oxford University Press, 1996. Discusses the physical effects of alcohol and caffeine consumption and suggests that some people become too reliant on alcohol to relax and on caffeine to give them energy. Braun discusses the cases of authors Ernest Hemingway, F. Scott Fitzgerald, and John Steinbeck—alcoholics who caffeinated themselves so they could write.

Edward M. Brecher, *Licit and Illicit Drugs*. Mount Vernon, N.Y.: Consumers Union, 1972. A thorough study of the history of drugs in the United States as well as an examination of the physical and mental effects of dozens of legal and illegal substances.

Janet Brigham, *Dying to Quit: Why We Smoke and How We Stop*. Washington: Joseph Henry Press, 1998. Mostly concerned with nicotine addiction, the book includes a chapter on smokers who also drink coffee and discusses how nicotine speeds delivery of caffeine to the body.

Stephen Cherniske, *Caffeine Blues: Wake Up to the Hidden Dangers of America's No. 1 Drug*. New York: Warner Books, 1998. The author, a nutritionist, makes a strong case for people to be wary of caffeine use. He also offers dozens of tips on how people can avoid caffeine and where they can find alternative products.

Frances Sheridan Goulart, *The Caffeine Book: A User's and Abuser's Guide*. New York: Dodd, Mead & Co., 1984. Complete assessment of caffeine as well as its benefits and risks; includes tips on how to survive the withdrawal symptoms and how to select caffeine-free alternatives.

Margaret O. Hyde and John F. Setaro, *Drugs 101: An Overview for Teens*. Brookfield, Conn.: Twenty-first Century Books, 2003. Covers issues surrounding the abuse and health effects of several drugs, including caffeine. Discusses how caffeine users can develop a tolerance to the drug and explores symptoms associated with caffeine withdrawal.

Cynthia Kuhn, Scott Swartzwelder, and Wilkie Wilson, *Buzzed: The Straight Facts About the Most Used and Abused Drugs from Alcohol to Ecstasy*. New York: W.W. Norton and Co., 1998. This book gives information about dozens of drugs, including caffeine. The authors outline the history of caffeine use and explain how caffeine travels through the body and affects the brain. The book also lists the caffeine content of several products and discusses health effects that heavy caffeine users may face.

Elizabeth Ann Nelson, *Coping with Drugs and Sports*. New York: Rosen Publishing Group, 1995. The author includes caffeine among the drugs that athletes often use and abuse; she points out the impacts on health that caffeine can cause if used in large quantities or in concert with other drugs, including painkillers and nicotine.

Jill Norman, *Coffee*. New York: Bantam Books, 1992. A brief history of coffee that also includes recipes for preparing unusual blends.

Mark Pendergrast, *Uncommon Grounds*. New York: Basic Books, 1999. An exhaustive history of coffee use in the United States and the world, tracing the evolution of coffee from its earliest consumption in the Middle East to the establishment of today's gourmet coffee bars.

Howard Schultz and Dori Jones Yang, *Pour Your Heart Into It: How Starbucks Built a Company One Cup at a Time.* New York: Hyperion, 1997. Schultz, the chairman and chief executive officer of Starbucks Coffee, tells how he built the chain into a corporation with more than $5 billion in annual sales.

Bennett Alan Weinberg and Bonnie K. Bealer, *The Caffeine Advantage.* New York: Free Press, 2002. The authors explain how coffee can be used to a consumer's advantage to stay alert, think straight, and compete in sports at a high level.

————, *The World of Caffeine: The Science and Culture of the World's Most Popular Drug.* New York: Routledge, 2002. The authors examine caffeine use over the years and provide assessments of the health risks and benefits of the drugs.

Periodicals

Barnaby J. Feder, "The Latest Mousetrap: Caffeine-Laced Spring Water," *New York Times,* May 6, 1996.

Beatrice Trum Hunter, "Some Health Effects From Caffeine," *Consumers' Research,* January 1, 1999.

————, "The Evolution of Chewing Gum," *Consumers' Research,* December 1, 2003.

Marianne D. Hurst, "Caffeine's Impact on Students Cited in Push to Curb School Drink Sales," *Education Week,* March 12, 2003.

Zachery Kouwe, "Here's a Jolt: Caffeine Exists Where It Often Isn't Expected," *Wall Street Journal,* June 10, 2003.

Judy Monroe, "Caffeine's Hook," *Current Health 2,* January 1, 1998.

National Public Radio, "Interview: Bennett Alan Weinberg discusses the discovery of caffeine, the significant amounts consumed daily, and the book he co-authored, *The World of Caffeine,*" Weekend Edition Saturday, September 8, 2001.

————, "Caffeine Consumption Linked to Miscarriage," Morning Edition, December 22, 1993.

Anne Neville, "Fill 'er Up: Coffee Is the Jolt that Fuels the Day for Local Caffeine Junkies Hot on the Trail of a Fix," *Buffalo News,* August 28, 2005.

Jeremy Pawloski, "Report Blames Caffeine OD in Mom's Death," *Albuquerque Journal*, November 30, 2004.

Charles P. Pollack and David Bright, "Caffeine Consumption and Weekly Sleep Patterns in U.S. Seventh-, Eighth-, and Ninth-Graders," *Pediatrics*, January 1, 2003.

T.R. Reid, "What's the Buzz?" *National Geographic*, January 1, 2005.

C.J.D. Sinclair and J.D. Geiger, "Caffeine Use in Sports: A Pharmacological Review," *Journal of Sports Medicine and Physical Fitness*, March 1, 2000.

Jim Stoppani, "Caffeine + Exercise = Fat Loss," *Joe Weider's Shape*, February 1, 2003.

Dana Sullivan, "Wake Me Up: A Cup of Coffee to Kick Start Your Day Won't Harm Your Health," *Real Simple*, December 1, 2004.

L. John Wertheim, "Jolt of Reality: Following the Lead of Elite Athletes, Teenagers Are Increasingly Juicing Their Workouts with Pills and Powders—Sometimes with Tragic Results," *Sports Illustrated*, April 7, 2003.

Duff Wilson, "A Sports Drink for Children Is Jangling Some Nerves," *New York Times*, September 25, 2005.

Internet Sources

AdvoCare International, "KickStart Kids." www.advocare.com /store/getProductDetail.do?itemCode=K2083&id=H.

Ari Bloomekatz, "Medical Experts Warn of Unhealthy Buzz-Touting Energy Drinks," *Seattle Times*, August 15, 2005. http://seattletimes.nwsource.com/html/health/2002430338 _healthenergy10.html

CBS News Early Show, "Kicking the Caffeine Habit," February 25, 2005. www.cbsnews.com/stories/2005/02/24/early show/living/ConsumerWatch/main676309.shtml.

Center for Science in the Public Interest, "Label Caffeine Content on Foods, Scientists Tell FDA," July 31, 1997. www.csp int.org/new/caffeine.htm.

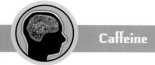

Consumer Reports, "Caffeinated Kids," July 1, 2003. http://www.consumerreports.org/cro/babies-kids/caffeinated-kids-703/overview.htm

Rob Cross, "Caffeine Use 'Bordering on Cheating': WADA," *ABC Premium News*, May 18, 2005. http://www.abc.net.au/sport/content/200505/s1371529.htm

Lauren Howard, "Fueling the Drive," *Decatur Daily*, Oct. 18, 2005. www.decaturdaily.com/decaturdaily/teenpage/0510108/fuel.shtml.

Steve Mraz, "Reporter's Notebook: Trick for a Caffeine Jolt Is far from Gourmet, But It'll Do," *Stars and Stripes*, October 4, 2005. www.estripes.com/article.asp?section=104&article=31191&archive=true.

National Coffee Association, "Caffeine Helps Keep Soldiers Vigilant and on Task," October 21, 2004. http://coffeescience.org/media/military.

———, "Science Will Change Our Perspective on Coffee, Says Expert." October 21, 2004. http://coffeescience.org/media/perspective.

National Public Radio, "The Coffee Break," *Morning Edition*, December 2, 2002. www.npr.org/programs/morning/features/patc/coffeebreak.

Linda Shen, "Campus Buzzing for Caffeine," *The Daily Tar Heel*, September 21, 2005, www.dailytarheel.com/vnews/display.v/ART/2005/09/21/4330d92879ed7.

Rick Telander, "The Big Enchilada: Tony Mandarich, a Top NFL Prospect, Is a Chowhound Who Chews Up Opponents," *Sports Illustrated*, April 24, 1989. http://sportsillustrated.cnn.com/2004/pr/subs/siexclusive/07/08/flashback.mandarich/index.html

Websites

International Food Information Council (http://ific.org/publications/brochures/caffeinebroch.cfm). This website includes information about the history, benefits, and health effects of caffeine.

The National Coffee Association (http://coffeescience.org). This group, formed to promote coffee consumption, has posted many scientific reports regarding caffeine use on its website. The reports, written by scientists and physicians, assess caffeine's effects on human health and its potential to fight Parkinson's disease, cancer, and other debilitating illnesses.

Neuroscience for Kids (http://faculty.washington.edu/chudler /caff.html). This website, maintained by the University of Washington, discusses the effect of caffeine on the brain and central nervous system in easy-to-understand terms. The website also includes information on the amount of caffeine found in various products and statistics about caffeine consumption in the United States.

INDEX

100

PICTURE CREDITS

ABOUT THE AUTHOR

Hal Marcovitz is a journalist who lives in Chalfont, Pennsylvania, with his wife Gail and daughters Michelle and Ashley. He has written more than seventy books for young readers as well as the satirical novel *Painting the White House*.